Praise for New Moves in Menopause

"Every once in a great while, you meet a magical person whose vibrant energy is completely infectious! Working with Maria as my menopause coach completely shifted how I see this stage of life. Maria has a rare gift for turning what feels like a challenge into an adventure and this book captures that magic perfectly. Reading New Moves is like having Maria on your team, guiding you through powerful explorations and helping you map a route to fitness and wellbeing that's refreshingly honest—and surprisingly fun! Her movement expertise, infectious energy, and creativity helped me confront hard truths and celebrate the adventures still to come. Now you can, too."
—**Halle Berry**

"Maria is one of the rare real ones. She writes with deep compassion, experience, and joy, taking women on a journey to learn not only to be their healthiest selves through midlife and menopause, but also their happiest. "
—**Selene Yeager**, host of the *Hit Play Not Pause* podcast and content manager at Feisty Media

"Maria is a bright light to follow during what can be a tough time for a lot of women. Her enthusiasm, wit, and actionable tips to not only survive but thrive in perimenopause and menopause is truly life-changing."
—**Wendi Aarons**, author of *I'm Wearing Tunics Now*

"*New Moves in Menopause* is a compassionate and practical guide to navigating menopause with confidence and clarity. Dr. Maria Luque brilliantly weaves together movement science, body respect, and real-world wisdom that gently challenges old beliefs while helping shape a more sustainable (and fun!) relationship with movement. It's exactly the kind of resource I'm excited to put into the hands of the women I work with every day."
—**Dr Jenn Salib Huber** RD ND, author of *Eat to Thrive During Menopause*

"Maria Luque is handing out permission slips to give ourselves a big old break, along with dishing out the kind of straight talk about movement and nourishment in menopause that we really need right now. I knew Maria was the real deal from the first time I interviewed her years ago, and that she was going to be a beacon for midlife women. She remains one of the most reasonable, upbeat, studied and experienced women in the modern menopause space. To the lucky, possibly lost-right-now lady who picks up this book: you will get to experience all that—and hopefully find your way from chasing perfection to self-connection along the way."
—**Ann Marie McQueen**, founder *Hotflash Inc*

"Maria shares her expert knowledge and shows readers how to apply it. She explains what's happening in your body, then offers practical ways to manage it, along with thoughtful guidance on how to talk to yourself along the way. This book normalizes menopause, helping women understand they're not falling apart, they are experiencing a natural biological phase of life."
—**Meredith Walker**, co-founder of *Amy Poehler's Smart Girls*

"In a world where it seems like everyone is telling women what they can and can't do, Maria invites us to bring passion and joy back into our lives. It's the reminder we all need that our bodies don't demand complex protocols or perfection to thrive—we can find a path to feeling great and living well that feels like play, not work."
—**Elizabeth Knight**, PhD, DNP, Integrative Women's Health Researcher

"As a physician who works with midlife women every day, I see how confusing and frustrating movement can feel during menopause. Dr. Maria changes that. She truly understands the menopausal woman and meets her exactly where she is, making movement feel doable and enjoyable, when many women feel out of sync with their bodies. This book is a practical, empowering guide whether you are just getting started, resetting your approach, or staying consistent with movement in this season of life."
—**Sarah de la Torre**, MD, FACOG, DipABLM

NEW MOVES IN MENOPAUSE

A Fearless Guide to a Stronger, Healthier, & Saner Midlife

MARIA LUQUE, PHD

with Robin Chotzinoff

New Moves in Menopause—A fearless guide to a stronger, healthier, and saner midlife

Fitness in Menopause, LLC
www.FitnessinMenopause.com

Cover photo by Cliff Watts
Cover design by Jessika Clarke
Edited by Robin Chotzinoff
Copy editing by Shelly Leuzinger

This book is for information and educational purposes only and is not intended to act as a substitute for medical advice or treatment. Any person with a condition requiring medical attention, should consult a qualified medical provider.

ISBN: 979-8-234-04165-4

Publisher: Fitness in Menopause

First Edition: May 2026

For my daughter Charlie
Because of you, I live with more joy, courage, and curiosity. Thank you for changing the
way I see life.

Acknowledgements

This book, and the wild, wonderful, occasionally chaotic journey behind it, would not exist without my village. My community, my friends, and my Fitness Fairies (you'll learn more about them in this book). You are my people, my hype squad, my "you've got this" when I absolutely did not feel like I had this.

When the path got dark, you showed up with flashlights. Every breakthrough, every 'aha!' moment, every victory has your fingerprints all over it.

You listened without judgment. You cheered without conditions. You redefined what family means to me.

I am grateful for every single one of you.

A very special thank you to Robin Chotzinoff, my co-author and the person who somehow made sense of everything swirling around in my head. The knowledge, the experiences, the very big and crazy ideas—you had the extraordinary gift of taking all of it and helping me shape it into something I am deeply, genuinely proud of.

You asked the tough questions. You pushed me to go deeper. And when the words finally landed on the page just right, it was because of your remarkable ability to turn my whirlwind into clarity. Thank you.

Chapter 1: Hello

Every New Year's Eve, I sit down with a stack of magazines, scissors, glue, and a blank poster board and begin my vision board. It's one of my favorite rituals. There's something almost magical about cutting out words and images and assembling them into a collage that represents my hopes for the new year. It's not just a fun art project; it's a map of where I want to go and who I want to become.

Looking back on twenty years of vision boards can be a surreal eye-opening experience. My earliest boards were loud and chaotic, plastered with words like "WIN" and "ACHIEVE," glossy images of chiseled bodies, luxurious cars and sprawling mansions. Those old boards almost seem to be yelling at me, which, truth be told, is perfectly in line with who I was back then—confused, unhappy, and desperately trying to force myself into a mold I thought would make me happy. I was using my vision board to represent the life I thought I was supposed to want.

Fast forward to now. My recent vision boards look very different, but not because of any conscious decision I made. In fact, I was surprised by the dramatic changes I saw—luxurious cars replaced with photos of where I picture myself hiking, using my own internal engine to take myself on an adventure. No high-tech home theaters, but a cozy reading nook with overflowing bookshelves. No 'ideal' bodies—in fact, no bodies at all, just images of what my body might *experience*: traveling to Australia and Japan (two of my bucket list trips), dense, peaceful forests and lots of cartoon animals—a happy ferret driving a tiny car!

My vision boards are no longer a reflection of what I think I *should* want, but an honest expression of who I am and what I value. They're about creating a life that feels good on the inside, not just one that looks good on the outside. Back then, I was chasing happiness. Now, I'm cultivating it.

Reviewing my vision boards reminded me that who we are at 20 is not who we are at 40, 50, or beyond. If we cling to the same goals, the same ideas of success, or the same approaches to movement, nutrition, and mindset, we're setting ourselves up for frustration and disappointment. Life is dynamic, in other words, and so are we.

My promise to you

If you're reading this, chances are you're navigating the choppy waters of menopause. Maybe you feel overwhelmed, confused, or frustrated by all the noise out there—the programs promising quick fixes, the miracle pills for belly fat, the cult-like devotion to high-intensity workouts, and the pressure to look like you're 25 again.

Of course you're overwhelmed! In one generation, we've gone from not discussing menopause in public to an overload of "information," not much of it credible. And yet there's plenty to learn about and from this natural human transition. So if you're tired of panicking about aging, if you want more depth and less surface, if you're ready to redefine what your body and life can be—well then, this book is for you. I hope to show you a new way of thinking about your body and how it moves—a way that prioritizes strength, self-discovery, and aliveness.

I'm your guide. Allow me to introduce myself

I grew up in Zweibrücken, a small town in Germany, where movement wasn't scheduled or tracked, but simply a way of life. Even in bad weather, I rode my bike to school, because it was way more fun than taking a crowded bus. My parents, both born in Spain, gave us a Mediterranean lifestyle—not just the food, but the constant, natural movement and strong sense of community. On weekends, my friends and I would map out bike routes in nearby France, pack up tents, and pedal through the countryside, laughing and challenging each other to race along the trails. At night, we'd eat and sleep under the stars.

Most Sundays, my family participated in a Volksmarsch—a "people's walk." It wasn't a race, but a fun, non-competitive hike through the countryside with family, friends, and friends-to-be. My parents, aunts, and uncles chatted while we kids chased each other through the woods. At the end of the trail, we'd be greeted by the delicious scent of bratwurst on the grill and the clink of beer glasses.

In high school, I developed a passion for handball, a sport that gave me my first taste of teamwork and physical grit. Practices were intense, but so were the post-game celebrations. And I played countless impromptu soccer games during school recess, with no scoreboard and no coach, just a ball and a group of kids with twenty minutes to spare for pure exhilaration.

After graduating from college with a major in Linguistics and Translation (Spanish, German, English), I married an American GI and moved to San Antonio, Texas, where I joined the U.S. Air Force. My roles varied widely: I started as an accountant and eventually worked my way up to lead the Commander's Action Group at Vandenberg AFB. I also served as a Sexual Assault Prevention and Victim Advocate, and I eventually became the base's Fitness Program Manager. That's where I really discovered the power of movement, both physical and emotional, as a way to heal and strengthen.

It may surprise you to know that I didn't step into a gym until I moved to San Antonio, where it wasn't as easy to just walk or bike or go for a hike. Feeling lost and out of place, I joined a big box fitness center. I wasn't used to working out inside, let alone in such a shiny, indoor setting, with machines lined up in rows and people monitoring themselves intently in the many floor-to-ceiling mirrors. I eventually realized that they weren't moving for joy, but to change how they looked.

In the beginning, I loved the energy of it all, the feeling of showing up, of being part of something. But slowly, without even realizing it, I started absorbing the same messages. Before I knew it, I wasn't just observing, I was part of it. What started as a simple desire to move morphed into something much more complicated, a desperate need to change my body—and I have to admit that I loved those changes, at first. I loved pushing myself, adjusting the formula, and seeing "results." Looking back, I see how unhappy and trapped I felt, and how strength training promised control—over my body, my time, and my energy. But control was an illusion. Instead of the mastery I hoped for, I developed body dysmorphia, convinced that no matter how strong I got, it was never enough. It didn't help that the more I changed my body, the more compliments I got.

A few years later, during a military field exercise, I dislocated both shoulders and damaged my spine from neck to lower back. Recovery wasn't quick or easy. It took months just to heal, months more to become active again. I had to learn to slow down and listen to my body, not to push it through pain. That frustrating, humbling, and at times heartbreaking, process forced me to build a new relationship with my body, one based not on how hard it could work, but on how well it could heal, adapt, and simply *be*.

In 2006, I separated from the military, moved to Austin, launched a personal-training business and began earning my Master's in Health Education, and later my PhD in Health Sciences.

I also found myself coaching a low-cost neighborhood fitness class. This small group, mostly women, got to know each other during circuit training sessions on a sun-baked driveway, at every season of the year. We became close friends, as close as family. Two decades later, the Fitness Fairies are still going strong. To this day, the bond we built through movement (and gossip, and real, human connection, including all the ups and downs) is one of the most rewarding parts of my journey.

At this point, I've been in the fitness field for more than twenty years. I've worked with clients from all walks of life, learning just as much from them as they have from me. In the beginning, I was a hardcore trainer who believed in giving my clients exact instructions and staying on top of their progress toward their stated goals. My job, I thought, was to tell people exactly what to do—to hand out the plans, the reps, the rules. But I began to realize that fitness is about much more than following instructions. It's also about tuning in, both to science and to our own bodies.

It was my work with clients—and hearing their stories—that inspired me to focus my doctoral research on menopause and physical activity. Doctors didn't have the answers these women were looking for, and when they consulted less traditional sources, the information they found was either a strange mix of high school biology class and miracle cures or flat-out fear-mongering.

I saw how they struggled. Not just with hot flashes or fatigue, but with feeling like strangers in their own bodies.

A longtime client who'd always been active couldn't recognize herself in the mirror. Her body composition began to change. As often happens, she gained weight, most notably in her midsection. Her confidence began to crumble—she went on (and off) diets obsessively and kept trying to force herself into more hours of training. Obviously, this wasn't "working" for her, but she blamed herself, because. . .that's what people do.

A close friend experienced such severe menopause symptoms that she couldn't sleep through the night. She felt completely drained of energy, but continued to beat herself up for not being able to work out at her usual pace and intensity. She felt as if a part of herself was withering away.

These two examples clarified something for me: there had to be a way to use movement to support bodies instead of fighting against them, to help women feel better instead of adding to their stress.

And the frustrating part? The research was—and still is—limited. It often raises more questions than it answers. The word "osteopenia," for example, is a term coined in

1992 by a World Health Organization working group. It's defined as a loss in bone mineral density below normal levels. Almost overnight, it seemed, so many of my clients were being diagnosed with mild bone loss, and they were terrified. Yet none of them were told what to do about it!

I began seeing ads and posts about extreme solutions aimed at menopausal customers—fasting, juice cleanses and anti-aging treatments that promised to turn back time, but at what cost? Hormones were either demonized as dangerous or glorified as the ultimate cure-all, with little nuance in between. By this time, as I entered perimenopause, I began asking myself *what's missing in all of this?*

The answer: A real conversation about **quality of life**. Not about how to make menopause disappear, but how to come to terms with it. If they're lucky, I thought, women will spend a third of their lives in menopause, so why isn't there more emphasis on how to live those years with strength, confidence, and joy?

***

I'm still a fitness trainer, but now I'm also a **menopause coach**—yes, that's a real thing, if a relatively new one. Serendipitously, my Austin clients are exactly the right age for my services, and we just keep aging and evolving together. In the past year, I was invited to join ReSpin, the startup Halle Berry created to change the conversation around menopause, which introduced me to a whole new group of clients, including Halle Berry herself. Now I'm her menopause coach!

Some of the most powerful transformations came not from lifting the heaviest weights or losing the most inches, but from women who learned to show up for themselves, compassionately, even when their lives grew messy and chaotic. Who realized that small, messy, imperfect actions still count, and that consistency beats perfection, every time. I've watched women walk away from workout programs that, for whatever reason, didn't inspire them, and replace them with routines that fit their real lives.

I'm in perimenopause myself, bringing my own struggles, challenges, and lessons to the table. And just so we're clear—I do struggle, because I'm human. As far as I'm concerned, we're all in this together.

One of my biggest battles? I'm a recovering exercise addict—and I feel strongly about calling it what it is—an addiction. Addictions don't make you happy, no matter how hard you chase them. Worse yet, exercise is supposed to be good for you, and that can really mess with your head. I'm still learning how to walk the line between a healthy and toxic relationship with movement, but I'm headed in the right direction.

I had to experiment with new moves, not just in how I trained, but in how I thought about movement. I had to unlearn the no pain/no gain mentality and replace it with something softer, wiser, and far more sustainable.

That's what inspired me to rebrand, from **Fitness in Menopause** to **New Moves in Menopause**. I envision New Moves as being about moving our bodies, but also about how we move through life. The New Moves approach values curiosity over control, compassion over comparison, and ongoing adventure over perfection. When we start seeing movement, and menopause, through that lens, it's no longer about fighting change. It's about learning to *move with it.*

You'll notice I use the word "movement" a lot—more often than "exercise," "fitness," and "workout," which often have connotations of rigidity, unrealistic standards, and shame attached. I want women to have a fresh start, which is what I think movement" gives us. Also, this is a book about New Moves, so how about we just . . . move? That could mean a lot of different things.

So, what am I offering you?

Think of this book as one of those old-school maps—creases, coffee stains, and all—leading you through winding roads, hidden detours, and unexpected discoveries. There's no single path, no pre-established directions. Instead, you get to explore, charting your own course based on what movement, self-care, and mindset mean to you. Some routes may feel familiar, others might take you somewhere new, but every step gets you closer to a version of yourself that feels strong, confident, and at home in your body.

How will we get there? (How to read this book)

Together, we'll explore how education, movement, nutrition, and self-care can transform your menopause experience. We'll also unlearn some of the messages and mindsets that have quietly shaped how we see ourselves—many of which have never served us, or simply no longer fit the women we're becoming.

We'll challenge the idea that smaller is always better, that rest is something we have to *earn*, or that strength training will make us *bulky*—as if muscle were something you accidentally scooped too much of in the grocery store's bulk-foods aisle. (News flash: the only thing that accumulates that quickly is laundry!) We'll question why we've been taught to fear aging instead of celebrating its freedoms. And we'll ditch the guilt that sneaks in when we choose ourselves—whether that's saying no to a workout because we need rest or saying yes to a long walk with just the right audiobook, not because it's *good for us*, but because it *feels good*.

Here's how this book is organized:

Chapter 1: Hello

Chapter 2: Menopause 101
What's happening, why it matters, and why you're not losing your mind (even if it feels like it sometimes).

Chapter 3: Who the Hell Am I Now?
Forget the old labels. This is about reintroducing yourself—to yourself.

Chapter 4: Body Image
Less fighting, more befriending. It's time to see your body in a whole new light. Desire, connection, and why your body's story isn't over (it might just be getting interesting).

How the Explorations work

Throughout the book, you'll encounter self-discovery prompts and exercises. You may have some experience with detailed goal setting, complete with deadlines, motivational mantras and a strong sense that if you don't psych yourself up, you'll fail. This is not that! Instead, I encourage you to take your time, engage your imagination, and give yourself time to evolve. These explorations are not supplementary—they *are* the journey. The insights you uncover by working through them will become the foundation upon which everything else is built. The questions may sometimes feel simple, but readers who answer them fully and mindfully tell me that's where the real breakthroughs happen. What you write, doodle, or even struggle to articulate on these pages will help you actively rewrite your story. That's not busywork. That's the whole point!

So while I would never dream of telling you what to do (okay, maybe just this once), I encourage you not to skip past them or promise yourself you'll come back later—we both know how that goes! Think of these explorations as an invitation to develop your own new moves.

I've added sample answers on the first page of each exploration, to give you a sense of how other women responded. The next pages are left wide open for YOUR answers.

You don't need the perfect answer, the uninterrupted schedule, or even the right pen—in fact, you can (and should!) assemble a healthy supply of colored pencils, erasers, and any other art supplies you enjoy using. You have my permission to make a mess on the page!

What this book isn't

A quick solution. If you're after a "flatten your belly in 5 days" crash course, this isn't it. No gimmicks and no promises you'll wake up a new person by Monday. What you *will* find is a real opportunity to roll up your sleeves, get a little messy, and uncover what happens when you stop trying to "fix" yourself and start partnering with your body instead. Some questions might poke at spots you'd rather leave undisturbed—but growth isn't supposed to feel like a spa day. It's more like planting a garden. You'll get dirt under your nails, mutter a few choice words when squirrels eat your tomatoes, and have a thousand opportunities to question whether you're even doing it right . . . until one day, you realize you're surrounded by the kind of beautiful, imperfect blooms that make every messy minute worthwhile.

A collection of proprietary miracle cures. Everywhere you turn, someone's promoting a shiny "fix" or a "hack" for what is, let's be real, a completely natural life transition. Menopause isn't an illness, it's not a medical condition, and it's definitely not a random collection of flaws that needs correcting. I'm not saying menopause doesn't come with challenges—of course it does, and you have every right to improve your quality of life at this time. But you're not broken. And anyone trying to convince you otherwise is just cashing in on your doubt.

A manual for how to regain control. In fact, if that's what you're chasing, you might find parts of this book a little . . . uncomfortable. I get it—women who've been successful at controlling their bodies through nutrition and exercise often have the hardest time with menopause. When things start shifting, their first instinct is often to double down, grip harder, and pour even more energy into discipline and willpower. I empathize with the longing behind it—the ache to hold onto what once "worked." I know how seductive—and how exhausting—it can feel. For many years, I clung tightly to the illusion of control, and all it did was drag me down a path of disordered eating and exercise addiction. So I'm not offering you more hustle. I'm offering ways to build trust, flexibility, and the kind of strength that doesn't vanish when life throws you a curveball.

A structured program that promises to take you neatly from Point A to Point B. Nothing wrong with those—and let's be honest, many of you could probably wallpaper a room with certificates from all the programs you've already crushed. But this is going to be different. Perhaps a little deeper.

Strictly a fitness book. To be clear, I *love* fitness. It's my bread and butter, the peanut butter to my jelly, and yes, I've spent years helping women move, lift, stretch, and build serious strength. But there's much more to New Moves than workouts, routines and obsessing over step counts, reps, or whether your fitness tracker gives you credit for "closing all your rings" today. Fitness is absolutely part of what we'll talk about, but it's not the *whole* story. I want us to think about movement in a bigger, wilder, more adventurous way that includes strength *and* flexibility, including the mental kind. We'll practice starting each day free of yesterday's judgments. We'll explore the kind of movement that feels less like atonement for your sins and more like your own brand of self-care and fun.

Menopause isn't easy (I won't lie), but it can be managed

Yes, it comes with physical symptoms—but it also comes with opportunities. Let's go!

Exploration: Permission Slip

Give yourself 15–20 minutes, ideally in a low-pressure setting. Gather your kit: a blank piece of paper, a journal, a notebook—as opposed to a laptop or phone—and one or two handwriting instruments—pens, pencils, whatever appeals. Feel free to break out colored pencils and/or markers. An eraser is nice too.

Think about what you hope this book might help you achieve, accept, grapple with, or . . . . Make some notes—whether neat and organized or messily scribbled makes absolutely no difference to me! Example:

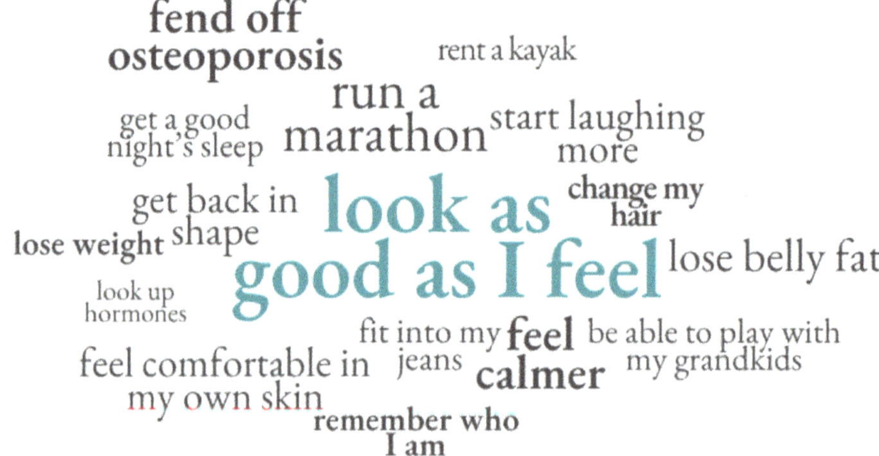

YOUR NOTES:

Exploration: Permission Slip

Just for a minute, pretend that discipline, time management, fear, confidence, hard work, and all those other common motivators have vanished from the face of the earth. Especially guilt. Kiss it goodbye. Now, give yourself written permission to go after what you want. Important: Don't think about how this would work in the real world. Just give yourself permission.

I GIVE MYSELF PERMISSION TO

- *get really, really sweaty*
- *stop dyeing my hair*
- *hire a babysitter/housekeeper/helper to free up time for myself*
- *stop worrying about protein*

My Own Most Recent Permission Slip:

- *I give myself permission to slow down when I need to, even if the voices in my head keep telling me to go and do more.*
- *I give myself permission to celebrate my body without apology.*
- *I give myself permission to choose happiness, even when life feels messy and out of control.*

Post your permission slip somewhere close—the fridge, above your desk, in your wallet. It's a powerful document. You have my full permission to do this as many times as you want.

Exploration: Permission Slip

Your turn...

Chapter 2: Menopause 101

"The menopause transition (perimenopause) and menopause that happen at the expected time are not diseases. This doesn't mean people don't have symptoms that might need to be treated, but menopause is not a medical condition because we expect the ovaries to decrease estradiol production. If menopause is a disease, then puberty must be one as well, and of course, it isn't."

—Dr. Jen Gunter

I remember my first real symptom of menopause clearly: anxiety. It hit me without warning, like a wrecking ball—just this sudden feeling that something was dramatically off. My heart raced for no reason, I'd wake up in the middle of the night filled with dread, and worst of all, I questioned myself constantly. *Why* was I overwhelmed? What had I done that made work, parenting and life—all meaningful activities I once took in stride—so challenging? There were no obvious clues, no night sweats or missed periods, to tell me that hormonal shifts were quietly rewriting the rules of my body and mind.

Years of menopause research sat in my head, yet anxiety blurred the obvious. Tracking my symptoms finally helped me connect the dots—I was in perimenopause. That's when I booked an appointment with my primary care doctor, and because I already knew which questions to ask, I was able to get the care I needed. I'm grateful for that head start—most women enter this maze without a map.

The same thing was happening to my clients. Symptoms of the menopausal transition seemed to be showing up everywhere I looked. Some were dramatic.

In the middle of a major presentation on stage, one of my clients felt the onset of a sudden, heavy period. Within minutes, blood had soaked through her pants in a very visible way.

A different client noticed something almost laughably small: the word "statistics"—which she'd used daily, for decades—suddenly slipped her mind, mid-meeting.

She brushed it off as stress, but a week later, "spreadsheet" disappeared. Then whole sentences began to feel as fuzzy as half-developed Polaroids—visible, but faint and grainy. She compiled a sticky-note sheet of "missing nouns" on her laptop, worried she was losing her edge or approaching early dementia.

A third client told me she would sometimes lock herself in the closet to cry for no apparent reason.

Despite how often they're reduced to punchlines, those symptoms are no joke. They can be disruptive, embarrassing, and often isolating, especially when you first become aware of them. Whether you're desperate for temperature regulation or weepy for no reason, at some point you'll find yourself wondering *what on earth is going on with me?*

Well, menopause. A complicated process. But knowledge is power, and whether you're just starting this journey or well into it, my goal is to help you make sense of it. So let's get into the basics.

The three (hard-to-pin-down) stages of menopause

- **Perimenopause**—when hormone levels start fluctuating and symptoms begin to appear. Menstruation continues, sometimes erratically and/or sporadically. While the average onset of perimenopause happens in the early to mid-40s, there are wide individual variations, from the late late 30s to early 50s.

- **Menopause** is more of a day than a stage—it's when you've gone 12 months without a period. The average age of natural menopause in the United States is approximately 51, with modest variation by race and ethnicity. Black and Latina women tend to experience menopause slightly earlier, while Asian women often reach menopause at the same age or somewhat later than white women.

- **Postmenopause**? That's everything that comes after that day known as menopause. In other words, the rest of your life.

You'll notice I use bullet points to describe the stages of menopause, but that's not how it works in real life. There's no neat list to check off; no calendar reminders that pop up on your phone. Menopause isn't a switch that flips on overnight. It's more as if your reliable Wi-Fi network begins glitching. Sometimes for minutes, sometimes for hours. Some days, you wonder if you imagined the outages because your Smart TV, laptop and thermostat are operating just fine. As time goes by, though, this unpredictability becomes your new reality.

People describe having gone "through" menopause, of women who "sailed through" or "barely made it through" menopause, as if everyone in the middle of this transition were headed toward a clearly marked exit. That's not really how it works. For most women, somewhere between 2 and 5 years after the final menstrual period, hormonal fluctuations settle at a lower, but steadier, level, and the body continues to adapt to what has become the new normal. Let's not forget this isn't your first time navigating a hormonal upheaval. You've done this before—maybe without even realizing how much was going on in your body behind the scenes. Puberty, pregnancy, postpartum, high-stress seasons . . . your hormones have been through plenty!

Hormone testing

Because of how much hormone levels fluctuate during the transition, hormone testing isn't the golden ticket some hope it will be. A single test can't tell the full story. Levels of estrogen, progesterone, and other key hormones can swing dramatically within a single day in perimenopause. That's why symptom tracking and understanding the *overall* phase you're in (such as perimenopause or postmenopause) is much more useful than chasing numbers.

That said, testing can be helpful in specific situations. For example, since women without a uterus don't have a final period that marks the milestone of menopause, blood tests can offer them some clues. Dr. Sarah de la Torre, double board-certified women's health and hormone expert, says, "Hormone testing comes in various forms: serum (from blood draws), saliva and urine. Each tell us something different and none are perfect. If the patient is telling me something different than what the lab reflects, I need to dig deeper to figure it out."

At the end of the day, it's less about pinpointing your exact location on the map and more about knowing what's happening in your body and what's ahead.

Welcome to menopause, brought to you by hormones!

Um, what *is* a hormone? Skip the following if you remember it from past biology classes (or present employment), but for the rest of us, this description from Janet Raloff (2017) is pretty good:

> All of us started as a single cell. Along the way, that cell divided and morphed in very individual ways. Some of us may have ended up short or tall, dark skinned or light, clever or slow, night owls or early birds. Scientists like to attribute most of those traits to inherited genes. But much of the work in crafting the traits that make each of us unique is performed by a family of chemicals known as hormones.

> Various tissues of the body secrete hormones into fluids, like blood. From there, the hormones travel far from the place they were made until they reach cells that read the chemical as an instruction.

> That hormone might tell the cell to grow—or to stop. It might direct a cell to change its shape or activity. These instructions might cause the heart to pump more rapidly or signal hunger to the brain. Another hormone might let you know that you're full. One hormone latches onto sugar in the bloodstream and then helps ferry that sugar into cells to fuel their work. Yet another might tell your body to burn some nutrients as fuel—or instead store their energy as fat for use at a later date.

Estrogen and progesterone

As we age, our ovaries gradually slow down the production of two key hormones: **estrogen** and **progesterone**. Clinically, the catch-all term **"estrogen"** encompasses three principal hormones—**estrone (E1),** synthesized mainly in adipose tissue and dominant after menopause; **estriol (E3),** produced by the placenta during pregnancy; and **estradiol (E2),** the highly potent ovarian estrogen that drives the menstrual cycle—so in midlife discussions, "estrogen fluctuation" is almost always shorthand for the dramatic rise-and-fall of estradiol.

Estrogen is the queen bee of your body, involved in everything from brain function to bone strength to heart health to skin elasticity. It even helps regulate body temperature and fat distribution.

Think of **progesterone** as a kind of weighted blanket for the brain. It typically rises in the luteal phase after ovulation. It eases anxiety and keeps stress from running wild.

Just so we're clear: hormone levels rise and fall with regular cycles throughout our lives—during puberty, pregnancy, postpartum, and high-stress times. Menopause, though, creates perhaps the most noticeable fluctuations.

During your reproductive years, progesterone and estrogen tag-team your menstrual cycle. Estrogen steps up first, helping to build and thicken the uterine lining in the first half of your cycle, preparing for a potential pregnancy. This is the follicular phase. Then, after ovulation, progesterone takes over, stabilizing that lining and preparing the body for possible implantation. This is the luteal phase. If no pregnancy occurs, both hormones drop, the uterine lining sheds, and voilà—your period.

But when estrogen and progesterone levels drop, things can get a bit chaotic. The ovaries don't retire gracefully. Some months, you might skip ovulation altogether and have no progesterone production and yet still have a period. Other months, estrogen might surge without enough progesterone to balance it out, resulting in anxiety, sleep disruptions, breast symptoms, irregular bleeding, heavier or lighter periods or skipped months.

Estradiol and progesterone don't snap to their new settings on the day after you've gone 12 months without a period. Research shows that estradiol and progesterone can stay somewhat erratic for another year or two before settling into a steady state.

The initial swings in estrogen levels cause many of the classic symptoms, such as hot flashes, night sweats, mood changes, and changes in body composition.

As progesterone fades out, you might notice more intense emotions, heavier or unpredictable periods, and for some women, a greater tendency to anxiety and depression.

Estrogen and progesterone aren't the only hormones shaping your experience. Let's meet the rest of the crew.

Testosterone often gets dismissed as the "male hormone," but it plays an important role for women, too. It helps build and retain muscle, supports bones, fuels sex drive, and generally adds that little extra spark. Declining testosterone levels are due more to age than to menopause itself, but their absence definitely contributes to feeling less strong, less energetic, and less . . . interested.

Think of **cortisol** as your built-in "get-stuff-done" hormone and your body's first responder for stress. It wakes you up, mobilizes fuel, and helps you handle stress, both life-threatening (being chased by a tiger) and modern-life frustrating (running late for a meeting.) Estrogen balances cortisol, smoothing out the big spikes by nudging the brain's stress thermostat (the HPA axis) to dial things back once the job is done. During menopause, estrogen's steadying abilities fade, so cortisol peaks can feel a bit punchier. But occasional surges are normal and even necessary. What matters is the daily rhythm, which can be influenced with the free basics—sleep, protein-rich meals, strength training, sunlight, and laughter—rather than dubious "cortisol-balancing" potions.

Think of **growth hormone (GH)** as your body's overnight renovation crew. While you sleep, it dispatches signals that patch and build muscle, persuades fat cells to release stored fuel, and nudges the liver to make insulin-like growth factor-1 so that your whole metabolic machine wakes up primed for action. What gradually makes this system less effective is not menopause but aging: average 24-hour GH output falls by about 12–15% with every decade after the mid-twenties, a change sometimes called the "somatopause."

The interaction between these hormones is what causes symptoms, which can come and go, show up in new ways, or even disappear for a while before making a grand re-entrance.

Physical changes

Attention: New body updates have been installed. Some features may not work as expected.

The physical symptoms of menopause tend to demand your attention. They show up in the fit of your clothes, your reflection in the mirror, your energy levels, even how you move through the world, forcing many of us to grapple with how enmeshed our self-worth may have become with our physical selves. As one of my clients said: "I feel like my body is betraying me." Many others have told me versions of the same thing. This sense of betrayal may feel familiar, if not exactly cozy.

I don't really need to describe **hot flashes and night sweats**—you'll know them when they happen. But they're often followed by **chills,** which can really keep you guessing at night. Yes, it's possible to sweat and shiver simultaneously.

Running on empty—by which I mean not just feeling tired, but that bone-deep exhaustion that makes you want to crawl into bed at 3 p.m., even if your day hasn't been particularly demanding.

Joint pain and muscle aches you can't quite explain. Maybe you're sorer after workouts, or not recovering as quickly from your favorite sports and activities. You can drive yourself crazy looking for an explanation, a treatment, a cure because, after all, something's wrong. Right? Yes, there is. There's actually a name for all this: *musculoskeletal syndrome of menopause.* It's not just in your head.

And of course there's **weight gain and/or fat redistribution.** Even with consistent eating and exercise habits, you may notice your body changing shape, especially around the belly, even if the number on the scale stays the same. Clothes fit differently. We'll dig into this more later, but for now, please realize: *this isn't your fault.*

Your **skin** may feel drier and itchier. Your **eyes** may feel dry, gritty, or more easily irritated. **Hair** can thin, especially around the crown, and/or develop a Brillo-like texture. **Breasts** can become unexpectedly tender. (There were days when I thought, *"Ouch! Touch these and you die!"*)

Peeing more often—or urgently—might become part of your new normal, along with **surprise leaks when you sneeze, laugh, or jump.** More frequent **UTIs** may show up too. **Vaginal dryness** is very real and very common, as is **discomfort during penetrative sex,** although it catches many women by surprise.

Mental and emotional changes

Overview: Your brain feels like a browser with 47 tabs open—and they're all frozen. *Those* changes.

Mood swings. One minute you're leading a high-stakes meeting, totally composed and in control—the next, you're trying not to sob over your inability to click to the next Powerpoint slide. One minute, you're feeling all sparkly on date night—the next, you're fixated on your partner's chewing. It's so loud!

Anxiety, especially when it represents a departure from your usual mood, can really throw us for a loop—both the sudden sky-is-falling episodes and those sneaky, daily thoughts of doom. As I said, this was my own personal first symptom, and I've since found out I'm not alone.

Depression can occur anywhere on the spectrum between foggy flatness and complete unraveling. Researchers have called the menopausal transition a "window of vulnerability" for developing a range of depressive symptoms. Either way, life seems beige, your motivation has packed up and left without notice, you're ever so weepy, you're saying "no" when you used to say "yes" . . . and scolding yourself for complaining, while you're at it. It's easy to downplay depression, to chalk it up to stress, overwork, aging, parenting, being single, being married or any of the many other non-easy parts of being alive. You may be tempted to do nothing; to hope it goes away on its own.

But here's a gentle suggestion—if these feelings persist daily for at least two weeks, check in with a professional. This isn't just my advice, it's a recommendation from The Menopause Society. Support is out there, and you don't have to navigate this alone.

Forgetfulness, brain fog, memory lapses. Such as that maddening moment when you walk purposefully into a room, ready to . . . what? You can't remember.

Such as the classic memory glitches: names, words, location of keys, appointments—poof! Gone. One of my clients nailed it when she said, "It's like my brain runs slower, but my worries move faster."

I definitely lose my train of thought. I'll be in mid-sentence, delivering a fascinating insight, when a winged creature swoops in, snatches the rest of my sentence, and flies away. (Yes, I fully picture this creature—a snarky little hybrid of fairy and cartoon crow, oversized reading glasses slipping down its beak, cackling as it hides my precious thoughts in a drawer labeled *"Things you'll remember at 3 a.m."*)

Understandably, many women worry that all of the above might be the beginning of dementia. These fears shouldn't be brushed off, but it is important to distinguish between dementia and brain fog. Simply put, dementia is forgetting ***what*** things are; brain fog is forgetting ***where*** things are. Think of it this way: with brain fog, the door to your memory is still there, and you still have the key, but you can't always find it in the moment. With dementia, the door and everything behind it gradually dissolve.

Changes in Libido. It's one thing to hear that a lower sex drive is "perfectly normal" in midlife. It's another to feel as if your sensuality has packed its bags and left the country. Higher sex drives are also possible. Either way, it's more accurate to say that menopause will *change* your libido, just the way it changes everything else.

Sleep disturbances. As in not being able to fall, or stay, asleep—along with all the collateral damage of trying to operate as a fully functional human without having really rested. On some level, you know that 2 AM is the wrong time to rethink your life choices and make imaginary grocery lists, yet that's what you're doing, night after night.

Now that I know what's happening, tell me how to fix it!

Once they understand what's happening, few of my clients are prepared to let menopause crash over them like the force of nature it is. In different ways, they'd all prefer some kind of plan of attack. I get it! I understand these desires to harness everything we've learned thus far, to go on the offensive, to *figure this out,* to work twice as hard. It's almost a rite of passage, this kick-menopause-to-the-curb response. But it's just that—a first step in a long-distance evolution.

"At 50, I read the Christiane Northrup book and then went out and bought $100 of worthless supplements at a big box vitamin store," says my client/friend Robin. "True story. For about three days I thought I had it figured out."

Another client spent an entire year on what I privately called "Operation Conquer Menopause." She burned through blogs and books, bought every supplement, and booked back-to-back appointments with any clinician who promised answers. A year later, she had nothing left but an impressive collection of contradictory advice and a feeling of having been gaslit. Then, just when she was about to give up, she met a doctor who actually listened—really listened—and offered a few practical tweaks. Her symptoms didn't magically disappear, but her stress did when she finally realized that menopause isn't a battle to win, but a stage to navigate, preferably with less chaos and more compassion.

A third client—I'll call her Superwoman—was determined to discipline her way through menopause. A lifelong competitive athlete, she was the kind of person who took every course, tracked every macro, and read PubMed studies as if they were bedtime stories. She knew exactly how to dial in her workouts and nutrition, and her body had always responded. In short, everything had always been under control—until it wasn't. Superwoman's body started to change, soften, thicken, and shift. She responded by doubling down on workouts, "cleaning up" her diet (which was already pristine) and telling herself she'd power through any and all symptoms like a champion.

But her body, specifically its new belly fat, didn't cooperate. And the harder she tried, the worse she felt, both mentally and physically. By the time I met her, her frustration had turned into outright shame. "I've never felt this out of control before," she told me. "I thought I was stronger than this."

"You are strong," I said. "But strength isn't just about pushing harder, it's also about knowing when to pivot."

Together, we began to unpack what was really going on. It wasn't just about fat gain. It was about identity. About control. About the belief that a shifting body was a symbol of failure.

It took time, but Superwoman stopped fighting her body and started listening to it. She learned to approach strength training in a new way, concentrating on what it gave her, as opposed to what it burned off. Her belly didn't disappear. But neither did she.

Remember, this menopause course isn't pass/fail. It's going to go on for a while. In a perfect world, your panic gives way to curiosity. So take a breath, and let's consider a few things.

The historical and cultural context, for instance. For the longest time, no one talked about menopause. Aging women were often feared, dismissed, or simply ignored. (Fun fact: throughout history, most of the women tried for "practicing witchcraft" were menopausal!) Many of our mothers and grandmothers went through this transition without mentioning it, because, after all, what clearer sign could there be that they were no longer useful? If they couldn't reproduce, what was the point? Better for women in midlife and beyond to fade quietly into the background.

Fast forward to today. Is it me, or is everyone suddenly talking about menopause? Between documentaries, books, podcasts, and entire wellness companies, menopause is having a cultural moment. For the first time, menopausal women are *more* visible, not less. We're pushing back against outdated ideas about what an older body can do, and research is finally starting to catch up. There's more respect for the challenges *and* the opportunities that come with this time of life.

But there's also a tidal wave of predatory marketing directed at keeping women's fears alive. The messages share a few common themes: *aging is bad, youth is currency, menopause is a disease/psychiatric disorder/character failing . . . but if you just buy this supplement/miracle serum/magical workout protocol/guru package, you (and a few lucky others) can turn back time.*

How's that working out for everyone? Hello?

If we're lucky, we have decades of life left to live. Midlife isn't the end of the story, but a whole new chapter.

A reminder: Menopause isn't an illness, but a natural transition whose symptoms can be managed.

If we're going to make the most of this transition, we must figure out how to manage it in a deeply personalized way, as well as how to maximize our quality of life, health and wellbeing. No two women will choose the same type of treatment—and that's exactly how it should be. Some may not need or want any treatment at all. Others will need a little extra help. None of it happens overnight. Most of us will have to let go of life lessons that no longer serve us.

Let's get into the treatment landscape.

Menopausal Hormone Therapy (MHT)

MHT is a powerful tool, clinically shown to be highly effective at relieving several key symptoms of menopause, including hot flashes, night sweats, vaginal dryness, sleep disturbances and bone loss. Like any tool, it works best when used for the right reasons, under the direction of the right clinician. The current confusion, fear, and mythology, both for and against MHT, is rooted in the Women's Health Initiative (WHI), launched in the 1990s.

One of the largest and most ambitious long-term studies ever conducted on women, the WHI was designed to evaluate the effects of estrogen and progestin therapy (E+P), and estrogen-alone therapy (ET), on the risk of cardiovascular disease, cancer, osteoporosis, disability, and poor quality of life in postmenopausal women. The original paper by the WHI investigators, concluded that "On May 31, 2002, after a mean of 5.2 years of follow-up, the data and safety monitoring board recommended stopping the trial of estrogen plus progestin vs placebo because the test statistic for invasive breast cancer exceeded the stopping boundary for this adverse effect and the global index statistic supported risks exceeding benefits." Panic ensued. Overnight, hormone therapy went from being seen as a standard, almost automatic, treatment for midlife women to something portrayed as dangerous, even deadly. We're still cleaning up that mess today. To this day, many still believe that HRT causes breast cancer. In fact, it's not so black and white.

The problem? The headlines didn't tell the full story—and the way the study was structured had major limitations.

Since then, many scientists have refuted and criticized the findings, including investigators from the original WHI study. The FDA recently removed the black box warning from hormone therapy. This reflects decades of updated research showing that for most healthy women, particularly those under 60, or within ten years of menopause, the benefits outweigh the risks.

However, if hormone therapy isn't right for you, there are now two non-hormonal, FDA-approved options for both hot flashes and sleep issues: fezolinetant (Veozah) and elinzanetant (Lynkeus).

"Alternative" hormone therapies

If you've spent any time online, you've probably been bombarded with promises to "balance your hormones, naturally" through supplements, diets, detoxes, breathing techniques or . . . something bad will happen.

If you're anything like me, you have a lot of questions, such as:

- What do these manufacturers mean by "balance?"

- Which hormones? (There are at least fifty identified hormones playing all kinds of roles in our bodies.)

- Is this a throwback to a time when MHT was known as "hormone *replacement* theory"—as if during menopause, women's bodies went into a kind of unnatural deficit, and only through replacement of what nature intended, but for some reason offloaded?, could women be made normal?

- Following that logic, are women in menopause hormonally "out of balance?"

- And what about *naturally?* Is there an *unnatural* way to balance hormones?

You can probably tell I don't take these products very seriously. Here's the thing—hormone levels fluctuate throughout our lives, not just in menopause. There's no such thing as optimal hormonal balance, or a level to strive for and maintain. Hormones can absolutely be used therapeutically during menopause, but they're not like furniture you can rearrange to make your house look better. They're part of a complex, dynamic system that constantly shifts based on things like age, stress, sleep, nutrition, movement, genetics—and, of course, menopause. So, when evaluating alternative hormone therapies, ask the same questions you'd ask when considering MHT.

- Which symptoms of menopause does this product claim to treat?

- Has it been researched? How and by whom? (individual testimonials and Yelp reviews don't count.)

- What are the potential risks?

New treatments will always be on the horizon, and it's exciting to see what's coming. But here's the truth: not every symptom can be *cured*. They can certainly be treated, managed, or even, sometimes, ignored. Some strategies will take trial and error, most require a commitment over time and some are ridiculously easy. All need to be personalized if they're going to help you, personally.

That said, I'll now contradict myself with some **gloriously unsexy advice that benefits all women in menopause: <u>CONCENTRATE ON ENOUGH!</u>**

As in,

ENOUGH NUTRITION—Chronic undereating stresses your body out. Try to include all food groups, **enough protein and fiber, healthy fats, and colorful plants**.

ENOUGH MOVEMENT—In other words, try to get some exercise every day, but don't kill yourself doing it. Think building up, not breaking down. We'll talk a lot more about this in Chapter 5.

ENOUGH SLEEP—Good sleep matters. Not to state the obvious, but bodies renew and repair themselves while resting. Figuring out how best to fall (and stay) asleep is important, especially if you're the kind of person who secretly thinks the desire to rest is either a sign of weakness or a character failing. I'm not the expert on this, but better sleep is a learnable skill.

ENOUGH CONNECTION with other humans, or mammals, or both. Research shows conclusively that loneliness and isolation are terrible for your health. So find your people (and/or your dogs.)

Exploration: Your Symptoms

Think about your experience of menopause so far–specifically, symptoms. Identify 3 to 5 symptoms/changes you'd most like to address. If you need a prompt, feel free to review the physical, mental and emotional changes on the preceding pages. Don't worry about whether the symptoms that matter to you most would make sense to a medical practitioner, therapist, or fitness trainer. You're the expert on you.

Example:
- I feel like menopause has changed my personality. I used to just GO FOR IT, but now I dither endlessly before taking any kind of risk, even a small one.
- Just diagnosed with osteopaenia–NOW WHAT?
- Can anything be done about night sweats?
- Everybody's talking about "metabolic health" instead of "weight loss." Are they the same thing? Because I've been gaining and losing weight all my adult life, and I'm starting to wonder why I keep trying to get back to that magic (low) number. I've heard it's harder to lose weight in menopause, not that it was easy before!
- My skin is soooooo dry.

YOUR LIST:

We'll return to this in a minute.

Managing, maximizing and triage

All symptoms are not created equal! One woman's intolerable hot flash is another's "well, it was getting chilly in here, anyway." Also, some symptoms come with an expiration date—declining noticeably around five years after menopause—while others can be expected to persist, to one degree or another, for the rest of your life. (Your skin is unlikely to regain its elasticity on its own, while night sweats tend to subside after a season.)

When considering what to do about symptoms, it helps to realize that some may be inconvenient or mildly annoying, but don't rise to the level of *Oh my god, make it stop!* That's what I mean by triage.

I'm definitely a little more prickly around my partner. Suddenly I don't like how she loads the dishwasher! But I've decided it's not all bad to communicate instead of stifling myself. If I get too pissy, I remind myself to deliver my message in a kinder way.

In recent photos, I was shocked to see what looks like a big, pink bald spot! At first, I panicked—went down a google rabbit hole of "styling thinning hair," best haircut for old ladies, etc. Social media heard me and sent ads for everything from medication to some bizarre tinted powder that you spray on your scalp—basically, female combover strategies. But I've never been a primper and thin hair isn't going to change that. So I deleted the offending photos and moved on.

Sure, I have brain fog. Whenever someone says, "Don't forget!" I say, "Oh, but I will, unless you help me remember."

You may feel differently about brain fog, however. Many of my clients find it distressing, if not downright scary. They're frustrated that it can't be erased in some permanent way. Instead, they've had to develop individualized strategies, some of them quite creative, such as:

- Turning their houses into sticky-note wonderlands.

- Stashing notepads in every room—because who knows where genius (or grocery lists) will strike?

- Downloading any memo app that feels like more like a game and less like a chore.

- Setting as many alarms (with as many different ring tones) as necessary, sometimes to that the point that their phone appears to be training for a NASA launch.

- Renaming Siri in order to find her when she's lost. ("Martha! Where are you?!")

- Adopting a failure-positive mantra, such as *Oh well, who cares?* Or *Silly me. . .* Or *Aw shucks, I guess I just compromised national security.*

So, how else does this managing of symptoms work in real life? Glad you asked. I'd like to illustrate my answer with a case study.

Everyone's favorite symptom: BELLY FAT

We had to talk about it sooner or later, right? In the "Ask Well" section of the New York Times, Alice Callahan consults a few experts:

> This is a physiological change that, unfortunately, really happens to virtually all women as we age," said Victoria Vieira-Potter, an associate professor of nutrition and exercise physiology at the University of Missouri. "It's not something you did," she added, or an indication that you're letting yourself go, so to speak.

> And in the words of Dr. Gail Greendale, a professor of medicine at the David Geffen School of Medicine at the University of California, Los Angeles:

> What worries me is that women who are trying to do right by themselves and keep up their exercise habits and eat a good diet may feel defeated" if their belly fat doesn't budge, she said. "They may be doing everything they can, and their central fat may just have a mind of its own.

> —*Alice Callahan, New York Times, Why Do Women Gain Belly Fat in Midlife (2022)*

As estrogen levels decline in perimenopause and menopause, a redistribution occurs as fat storage shifts from our hips to our waist. Even if your overall weight doesn't change much (although for many of us it does by at least 5-10 pounds), more of it tends to settle around the middle. In other words, part of the change is hormonal and programmed into our DNA, and not a personal failure. Understanding this shift can take some of the blame off our plates, and our shoulders.

—Dr. Jenn Salib Huber RD ND

The "meno-pot"—and the struggle against it—seems to be an equal-opportunity anxiety. Regardless of their weight, body-fat percentage, or fitness level, women are psychologically vulnerable to this extra belly fat. It appears out of nowhere, they tell me. (Like a process server at the door?) Never mind how it got there, make it go away!

There's actually a pretty straightforward explanation for the menopause belly. Estrogen has anti-cortisol properties. As estrogen decreases during menopause, so do its cortisol-fighting superpowers, and as our algorithms have told us, cortisol activity is responsible for increased belly fat. We've probably also read that cortisol is the "stress hormone." Does that mean less stress equals a smaller waistline? Not really. While I fully support stress reduction, it's not a magic belly-fat bullet. You can, however, incorporate these strategies:

- *Work out with weights to build muscle mass.* Muscle is more metabolically active than fat; with more muscle, your body will be more efficient at burning calories.

- *Stress reduction.* Just as your body will send very clear signs that it's experiencing stress, you can teach your body to chill out. Try yoga, Tai Chi, meditation—anything that fits the general heading of mindfulness. Taking just a few deep breaths can help more than you might think.

- *Get adequate sleep.* 7 hours at minimum, 9 if you possibly can.
As for what to do about belly fat itself, you still can't spot-reduce! You never could, and you can't start now. Also, belly fat is not a character failing—a fact the rest of the world seems to be catching up with. But that doesn't mean the belly fat troll won't pay you occasional visits. You might want to try:

- *Acceptance and debate.* As we age, various hormonal and metabolic factors usually conspire to add abdominal fat. This is true for almost everyone, short of people who've had significant plastic surgery. With age, waists tend to expand. Does this mean you're now officially unattractive? No. Does it "mean" anything? I don't know—maybe that you're human? If you think back on your life so far, you might notice that when it came to your body, change has been a constant. You went through puberty, perhaps pregnancy, maybe an illness; you were fit and less fit, your hair turned grey, you learned how to do something you couldn't do before or were no longer able to do something you loved. All thanks to your amazing, imperfect body. And there's more to your body than your appearance. And there's more to your appearance than the size of your belly, which is what it is.

- *Acceptance, cinematic version:* Oh, hello Belly Fat! I see you're back for another visit. Can I get you a cup of tea? Okay, please go ahead and vent! I'm sure you have oodles of *brand new insight* to share!

- *Staying (or becoming) active.* Menopause is no reason to slow down. It might even be a reason to speed up. The more active you are, the better you'll feel in your own skin. All of you will feel firmer, no matter the circumference of your waist.

- *Striving to eat a wide variety of healthy foods.* Not to make your meno-pot disappear, but because—is there a good reason *not* to eat in a healthy way?

- *Saying no to snake oil.* There is no secret hack for spot-reducing your belly through sweat or starvation. Supplements are completely unregulated, so be suspicious of extravagant claims of magical fat-melting. You cannot "cleanse" your body of belly fat, either.

- *A ridiculously simple solution*, such as: <u>If your waistband feels uncomfortably tight, get a different pair of pants.</u>

- *A substantially difficult, but perhaps worthwhile, effort*, such as: <u>Find a better place to put all the energy you've devoted to agonizing over belly fat. Take that persistent drive and focus, and use it to solve a more important problem.</u>

A few more **RIDICULOUSLY SIMPLE SOLUTIONS** for other menopause symptoms:

- Keep a small cooler full of wet washcloths on ice next to your bed. Use as required for **cooling down night sweats.**

- Dress in light layers. In case of **hot flashes**, remove one or two, or all.

- For **vaginal dryness or recurring UTIs:** Ask your OB-GYN about low-dose vaginal estrogen rings. (Estring (™) is safe even for breast cancer survivors).

- For **weepy mood swings:** Buy yourself a half-dozen bandannas. Use them to mop up tears. Wash, rinse, repeat.

Exploration: Maria's Managing and Maximizing

Get out that list of symptoms. For each item, answer these questions:
- What is the generally accepted wisdom concerning this symptom?
- Have you tried any of these ideas? What was the result?
- How could you apply acceptance to this symptom?
- Can you think of a ridiculously simple solution—or a big, complicated strategy?

Example:

Symptom:
I haven't gained an ounce but I hate these new fat deposits!

What is the generally accepted wisdom concerning this symptom?
Um, go on a diet? Do more crunches?

Have you tried any of these ideas? What was the result?
Discouraging!

How could you apply acceptance to this symptom?
I could realize that everything changes, including bodies. I could be grateful for this body I have and quit insulting it.

Can you think of a ridiculously simple solution—or a big, complicated strategy?
I could learn about dressing to highlight the part of my body I like and downplaying the ones I'm learning to accept.

Your turn...

Exploration: Managing and Maximizing

Symptom 1:

What is the generally accepted wisdom concerning this symptom?

Have you tried any of these ideas? What was the result?

How could you apply acceptance to this symptom?

Can you think of a ridiculously simple solution—or a big, complicated strategy?

Exploration: Managing and Maximizing

Symptom 2:

What is the generally accepted wisdom concerning this symptom?

Have you tried any of these ideas? What was the result?

How could you apply acceptance to this symptom?

Can you think of a ridiculously simple solution—or a big, complicated strategy?

Exploration: Managing and Maximizing

Symptom 3:

What is the generally accepted wisdom concerning this symptom?

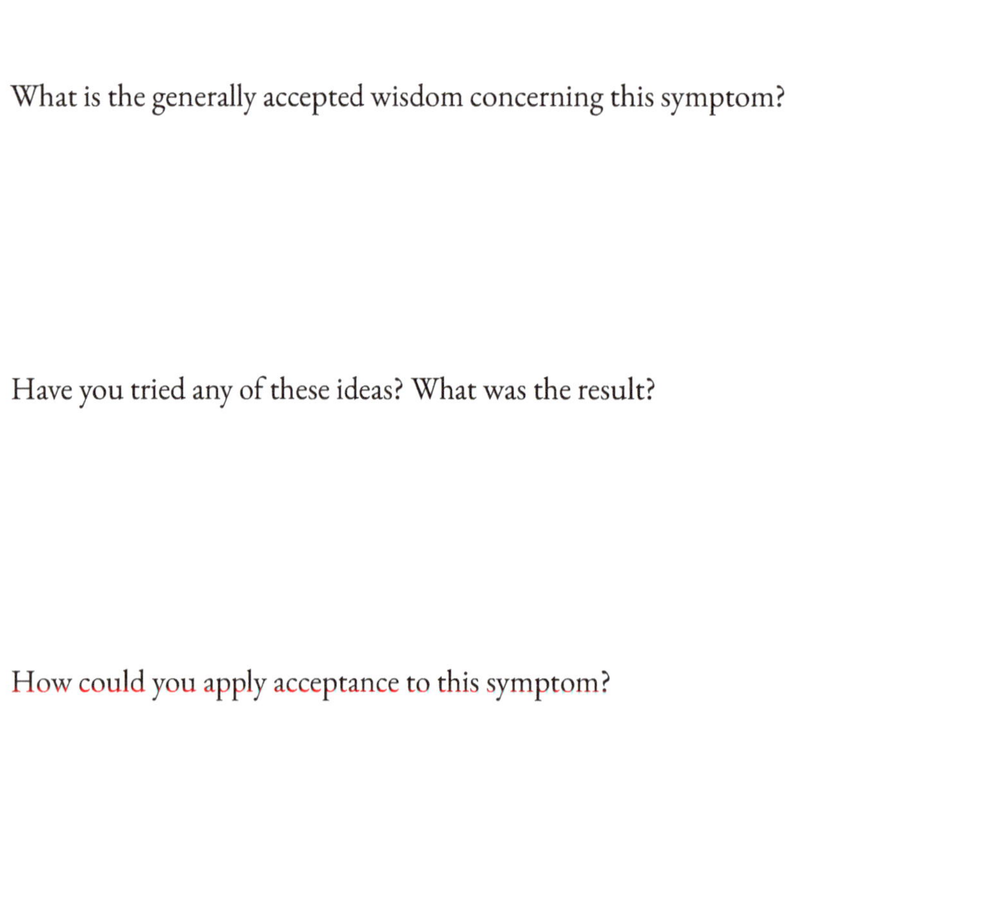

Have you tried any of these ideas? What was the result?

How could you apply acceptance to this symptom?

Can you think of a ridiculously simple solution—or a big, complicated strategy?

Exploration: Managing and Maximizing

Symptom 4:

What is the generally accepted wisdom concerning this symptom?

Have you tried any of these ideas? What was the result?

How could you apply acceptance to this symptom?

Can you think of a ridiculously simple solution—or a big, complicated strategy?

Exploration: Managing and Maximizing

Symptom 5:

What is the generally accepted wisdom concerning this symptom?

Have you tried any of these ideas? What was the result?

How could you apply acceptance to this symptom?

Can you think of a ridiculously simple solution—or a big, complicated strategy?

Chapter 3: Who the Hell Am I Now?

Warning: This chapter may cause unexpected clarity, spontaneous boundary-setting, and a deep desire to stop people-pleasing. Proceed with self-compassion—and snacks.

Making your way through menopause isn't like remodeling a house. You can't just call in an expert, make a checklist of necessary repairs, and hand the job over to the experts. There are symptoms you can address, absolutely—but maybe, just maybe, there's more to a satisfying life than relentless self-improvement. Who is this self, anyway? Maybe her priorities have shifted. Midlife is the perfect time to get reacquainted.

Rediscovering yourself is essential to growth, satisfaction and quality of life, especially in menopause. Not just for you, but for everyone who gets to experience the version of you that isn't hiding, shrinking, or running on autopilot.

All this requires work, but in my opinion, it's worthwhile. You may find it gives you energy to spare—enough to know yourself a little better. Or remember the self you used to know. Or learn more about the self you're becoming. Or all three.

That's what I mean by **new moves**—on your terms, in this chapter of life.

What will yours look like? That's what we're here to figure out. But first, some paperwork.

Here's your permission slip:

- To think for yourself.

- To take a few hours—or a few days—away from feeds that bombard you with aspirational imagery and expensive miracles, keeping you stuck in a world where you're only as good as your last age-defying humble-brag.

- To stop trying to win a game you never signed up to play. To learn a new one.

- You're not starting over. You're starting *from here.* You ready? Let's go.

***

Are you lost? Maybe that's too strong a word. Are you ever so slightly unmoored? Either way, join the menopause club, where we all feel that way, to one extent or another. The good news is you're not alone, and believe it or not, adventure lies ahead. But first, let's take a minute to process that *lost* feeling. It's almost as if you lost your self.

Where did you go? How did you get turned around? Look over the scenarios below and see if anything resonates:

- Some of us get lost in life's roles—wife, mother, helper, supporter, manager, person who smooths the bumps in the road so that her loved ones will have an easier ride. (I just raised my hand.)

- Some of us get lost in postponement—in being so busy taking care of other people and their latest crises that we never quite get around to taking care of ourselves.

- Some of us get lost in achievement—climbing the ladder, getting the gold star, following our ambition (or our bliss), discarding all unnecessary baggage as we go. Over time, our standards become more rigid and exacting. We stop checking in with our Selves.

- Some of us get lost in appearance-driven perfectionism—believing we need to look a certain way to be lovable, valuable, credible, even healthy. We're taught that if we age gracefully—if we stay thin, if we chase youth with enough Botox and green juice—we'll be seen as visible and valuable.

- Some of us get lost in the illusion of controlling our health, through clean eating, supplements, cold plunges, punishing physical activity—not because it feels good, but because we're chasing the seductive promise of outsmarting aging and illness. That if we do all the right things, we won't get sick, suffer, or die. Spoiler alert: We will.

- Some of us get lost in shame. Shouldn't we have succeeded more, in so many ways, by now? At this late date? We tell ourselves we should be fitter, better parents, better citizens, better bread-winners. We order ourselves to try again. Harder this time!

- Some of us get lost in soothing distraction—in filling time we could devote to real happiness with empty, but not unpleasant, filler. We all spend too much time doing nothing in particular on our phones, right? Which isn't so terrible, right? Right. But still. Mindless soothing activities—those dopamine bumps, those substances, that pleasure-chasing—can become addictions.

No wonder so many of my clients ask *When will I get back to normal? When will I get back on track?* But I can (and do) encourage them to think less about going back and more about moving ahead. Which is not to say that there's nothing worth rediscovering from our past histories.

However, when we start poking around in there, not everything we discover is treasure.

Cleaning out the fridge

You know that moment when you open your refrigerator and find a half-rotted lemon, a questionable hunk of cheese and a jar of pickles from 2019 staring you in the face? You planned to cook something nourishing—maybe even exciting—but now you'll deal with what's already taking up space.

That's where we are right now. Put on your big girl pants and get ready to throw out some mental garbage—the expired rules of a diet you hated, the congealed guilt over workouts you didn't do, the withered stalk of unmet expectations. (Oh, this is fun.) The freezer-burned sack of assumptions about how a woman is supposed to look and behave.

Let's just say it: we're all hanging onto some questionable items. If that metaphor's not disgusting enough for you, how about this:

Tuning out the Chatter

It's really hard to hear your own voice when everyone else's is so loud, and I do mean *everyone* else, because the chatter is broadcasting on every channel. It can sound like a helpful suggestion, a trusted expert, your own inner voice repeating something you heard three times today on social media, or:

- The fitness ads promising to "sculpt your menopausal belly"

- The influencer wellness routines that somehow require two hours, a $200 supplement stack, and zero children or real-life obligations

- The endless stream of articles, programs, and people telling you how to "live your best life"

- The friend who says, "You shouldn't eat bread. It's bad for you"

- The doctor who dismisses your symptoms because "it's just menopause," but tells you your workouts won't be effective unless you do them at night

- Your own distorted memories of achieving mastery over some part of yourself you thought needed fixing. Regardless of how much time you spent in this blissful state of control (it's usually less than you think) you're not there now, as the chatter is happy to remind you.

The chatter is sneaky. It's not a megaphone; it's more of an undercurrent. It's a weird mixture of exciting and red-flag-raising. It would be amazing, theoretically, to prevent heart disease, regrow my hair, rejuvenate my skin, melt my belly fat, and balance my hormones, but oh my God, I'd have to give up wheat (and all its wonderful relatives) and get yelled at in a dark room by a trainer half my age, and . . . calorie deficit? That old thing?

The chatter is neither backed by science nor imbued with common sense. For instance, the suggestion that you get your teeth and gums cleaned twice a year is not

Chatter. It may not be your idea of a fun time, but it's pretty much accepted as good advice. (If your dentist also suggested that a brand new "gleaming smile" would fix your every insecurity, that would begin to sound a little Chatter-y.)

So, here's your invitation: Start tuning out the Chatter, on purpose. This might mean unfollowing "aspirational" content that leaves you spiraling. It might mean asking yourself *Do I actually want this? Or am I just <u>supposed</u> to want it? Is this voice thinking about what's best for me? Do I feel more or less like myself when I'm listening to it?*

Whose voice is it, anyway?

The goal here isn't to isolate yourself, but to create space, so that your own voice—your preferences, instincts and wild ideas—can come to the surface.

Exploration: "Should" Detox (Example)

Pick 2–3 "shoulds" you've heard recently—from a friend, a doctor, a social media post, or your own inner critic. Ideally, pick shoulds with some real sticking power. Ones you can't stop thinking about. For each one, ask yourself four questions.

Example:

SHOULD:
I should stop eating after 6 pm.

1. Where did I hear this?
My skinny step-mom.

2. Why is it tempting?
If I did it, I could be skinny. Maybe.

3. Does it make me feel good or bad?
Bad. I love food and I hate to miss dinner.

4. If no one else's opinion mattered, would I *still* want to do this?
NOPE.

Your turn...

Exploration: "Should" Detox

SHOULD:

1. Where did I hear this?

2. Why is it tempting?

3. Does it make me feel good or bad?

4. If no one else's opinion mattered, would I still want to do this?

Now look at what you wrote.
- Where do you need a <u>hard stop</u>?
- Where might you be ready to say: "That doesn't work for me."
- What gets to stay, <u>because you chose it</u>?
- Optional: Do something small but symbolic. Throw out an old schedule. Delete a tracking app. Rip up a diet log. You get to make space.

Exploration: Maria's Passion Project

Here's how I filled out this exploration sheet.

Are there activities, pursuits, or passions you once loved but no longer do?

Passions (as a pre-teen)	What happened
Soccer during recess ☆	*Life doesn't have scheduled recess*
Bike rides with my friends to neighboring France to camp ☆	*Moved to the States, safety concerns, didn't have many friends when I moved here*
Going on long family walks surrounded by cousins, aunts, and uncles ☆	*Moved to the States and am not close to my family anymore*

Since the onset of menopause, what have you given up?

Discarded item	Foregone reward
Hourlong stints on a cardio machine	*Losing weight and fat*
Saying yes to activities I don't want to do just to please others	*Feeling like I was being a good partner, family member, friend for doing things with and for them*
Working out to lose weight	*Looking "good"*

Exploration: Maria's Passion Project

Are there activities, pursuits, hobbies, or passions you discovered (or rediscovered) since (approximately) the onset of menopause? Make a list on the left. On the right, add anything you've considered, but haven't yet tried.

Rediscovered / New Passion	Considered but haven't tried
Via Ferrata ☆ ✓	*Rapelling from a mountain*
Lazy beach vacations ☆ ✓	*Silent retreat by myself*
Racquetball ☆ ✓	
Bike rides ✓	

And now, answer these questions:

1. What did you learn about yourself from this exercise?

That I've been making a lot of positive changes to allow myself to do things I want to do and letting go of things I thought I should be doing or that had a misguided goal such as weight loss or pleasing others. I also noticed that I'm allowing myself to go back and revisit things (e.g., bike rides with friends) instead of just leaving them behind.

2. What surprised you?

I yearn for more alone time now when before it was all about being with others.

3. Who are you today? Answer using nouns (Example: adventurer, foodie, daughter, dolphin . . .).

Mom, explorer, teacher

4. Who are you becoming? Again, answer using nouns (Example: gramma, gymnast, butterfly, bookworm . . .).

Authentic, advocate, guide

Exploration: A Passion Project

Get out your kit–and don't forget the colored pencils! Are there activities, pursuits, or passions you once loved but no longer do? Include health- and fitness-related pursuits, but don't stop there—if you were really into puzzles or scrapbooking or triathlons, put it on the list. List your passions on the left. On the right, explain briefly why you no longer do this thing. Don't overthink! Just write whatever comes to mind.

Passions	What happened
Example: foreign travel	*The pandemic*

Exploration: A Passion Project

Since the onset of menopause, what have you given up? Make a list on the left.
On the right, write what reward this activity used to give you.

Discarded item	Foregone reward
Example: crossfit	*Competition and being pushed*

Exploration: A Passion Project

Are there activities, pursuits, hobbies, or passions you discovered (or rediscovered) since (approximately) the onset of menopause? Make a list on the left. On the right, add anything you've considered, but haven't yet tried.

Rediscovered / New Passion	Passions to try
Example: water colors	*Example: learning a new language*

Add a STAR next to something you want to keep doing (or wish you could do again). Important: Don't think about logistics, such as whether or not this activity is affordable, or realistic, or a "good" use of your time. Put a CHECK next to activities that just fit who you are right now, whether or not you're still doing them. CIRCLE items that are an example of positive change in your life—either from stopping or starting them. UNDERLINE to acknowledge something you feel good about having let go of, even if it wasn't easy. Think about this multi-colored portrait of yourself. Don't rush.

Exploration: A Passion Project

Let it all sink in. And now, answer these questions...

1. What did you learn about yourself from this exercise?

2. What surprised you?

3. Who are you today? (Answer using nouns, for example: adventurer, foodie, daughter, dolphin . . .)

4. Who are you becoming? (Again, answer using nouns, for example: gramma, gymnast, butterfly, bookworm . . .)

Chapter 4: Body Image

I'll just say it: if you think a fitness trainer never struggles with body image issues, you're wrong. In the fitness industry, the physical body holds immense value—it's almost like a business card. Appearance can seem more important than knowledge or experience, and it's common to get caught up competing with other trainers, on the basis of looks alone. The body dysmorphia that began in my twenties and persisted into my forties eased off, only to be replaced by the angst brought on by the hormonal changes of perimenopause.

So I'm quite clear that body image issues can't be overcome "once and for all," but rather managed over time. And by managing, I mean developing a kind and compassionate relationship with your body.

My shift toward real self-acceptance came at 41, when I had my daughter. Whether or not they were visible to anyone but me, the changes in my body felt dramatic and unsettling, and I was suddenly responsible for raising a new little person. If at all possible, I wanted her relationship with her body to be healthier than my own, and that meant taking a hard look at how I spoke and thought about myself.

I realized I'd been characterizing myself—and others—in physical, appearance-based ways, almost without realizing it. I didn't want my daughter to see me critiquing myself as I looked in the mirror. I didn't want her to hear me describe others that way, either, whether I was admiring them for being *ripped* or *fit* or *beautiful,* or judging them for being *unhealthy* or *overweight* or *unattractive.* It wasn't easy to break this unhelpful habit, but I was determined not to pass it down to my child.

She's 10 years old now, and I've come a long way in accepting my own, ten-years-older body. It's been through a lot. Between injuries sustained in the military and the natural wear and tear of life as a trainer, there are days when moving is tough and working out is a quiet conversation between pain and perseverance.

Some days, I decide on an easy walk with my dogs; other days, when my body feels more energetic, I push hard by doing a heavy workout, because I love the feeling of my muscles working. I've learned to give myself that space, to honor both kinds of days as part of the same story. My body deserves my respect; just as your body deserves yours.

Let's talk about how to get there.

***

Body image is the mental selfie you carry everywhere—an ever-shifting collage of how you *see* your body, what you *think* about it, and how you *feel* living inside it. Unlike the photos on your phone, this selfie updates in real time, filtered through culture, comparison, and the occasional carnival-mirror moment in a fitting room.

Body image is a multi-dimensional experience, not a dress size. It weaves together cultural messages, personal history, gender, race, age, ability, and a dozen other strands you don't see in the mirror. That's why *any* body can struggle with it.

The visual layer—"What I see"
Think mirror reflections, Zoom thumbnails, Facebook memories, or your reflection in a shop window.

The cognitive layer—"What I think"
This is the commentary track—everything from "My legs look strong today" to "Is that a *beard* hair?"

The emotional layer—"What I feel"
Pride, embarrassment, neutrality, delight—body image isn't just thoughts, but a collection of moods. Two women of the same size can feel worlds apart because emotion, not measurement, sets the tone.

The kinesthetic layer—"What I sense"

Often forgotten but crucial: How your body *moves* and *functions.* How it feels when you set a new weight record at the gym, or when too-tight clothes cut into your waist.

As previously discussed, the hormonal changes of menopause tweak all four layers of body image at once.

Here are some stunning facts:

- 60–89 % of mid-life women report some level of body dissatisfaction—even if they've never had an eating disorder or body dysmorphia.

- On average, girls internalize the thin ideal by age 6; in surveys, half of 9- to 10-year-olds have already tried dieting.

- Menopausal symptoms correlate *directly* with more negative body image perception.

- A 30-day mobile-tracking study found that even 10 minutes of scrolling "fit-fluencer" posts spiked body shame later the same day.

- Nearly 50% of American girls aged 13 report feeling unhappy with their bodies; this rises to 78% by age 17.

- 40–60% of elementary school girls are concerned about their weight or about becoming "too fat."

- Among middle-aged women (average age 55), 80.8% report dissatisfaction with their body image.

What we're up against

I'm sure I don't need to tell you that our culture worships *youthful, thin, and smooth.* Each birthday nudges us further from the air-brushed norm, keeping the "ideal" body just outside our grasp.

Negative body talk starts in kindergarten and cranks up to stadium volume during menopause—no hearing aids needed—with a few notably terrible stops along the way, such as the whole "bouncing back from pregnancy" narrative, or any message that puts a timestamp on our physiques.

A triathlete client was determined to reclaim her "2008 marathon body." But in 2008, she hadn't had two teens, a full-time job, or perimenopausal insomnia. When we reframed her goal from "reclaiming" to "re-imagining," her training became curiosity-driven instead of punishment-driven. She realized that her body—that awesome machine that had carried her through life, loss and growth—was still there for her, still going strong. The fixation on getting a particular version of it back now seemed kind of narrow.

How do we start to feel good inside the bodies we have *now*—not ten pounds from now, not post-cleanse, not once we finally "get back on track?" Well, negative body image is learned, as opposed to inborn, and we can chose to *unlearn it.* But what to replace it with? Is this a matter of ***just loving ourselves*** or ***body positivity?***

Not exactly. Those messages had their moment, encouraging us to embrace our bodies, imperfections and all. But they often ended up feeling exclusionary for those who struggled to muster love for their bodies during times of change—such as, you guessed it, menopause. The truth is, it's simply not realistic to feel good about your body 100% of the time.

That's where **body neutrality** comes in—a more compassionate and forgiving approach that allows us to acknowledge what our bodies can *do* rather than how they look. It's the middle ground between self-criticism and forced positivity. The goal isn't to adore your reflection; it's to stop your reflection from running your day. An example of reframing a body negativity comment to body neutral could be

Body-negative thought:
"I hate my stomach. I look disgusting in these jeans"

Body-neutral reframe:
"My stomach feels uncomfortable in these jeans. Maybe I'll choose something that fits better."

How to fight back

The quickest antidote to cultural crazy-making is small, deliberate moves that re-wire what you *notice, say,* and *do* about your body every day. Here are some messages and strategies that may help.

- **Health and quality of life *always* trump physical appearance.**

- Realize that **people come in all shapes and sizes.** The next time you find yourself in a crowd, take a long, judgment-free look at the variety around you. You can also **try this with dogs,** who come in an amazing array of breeds, sizes and physiques. Now observe yourself: are you more of a Great Pyrenees or a chihuahua? Does it matter which breed is popular right now? Would you expect a mastiff to diet down to greyhound size?

- Pay attention to **what your body can do, as opposed to how (you think) it looks**. You might feel silly, at first, but start a list of everything you couldn't accomplish *without* your body. If you've been alive more than a few decades, allow yourself to be amazed at how many feats of transportation, reproduction, survival, and fun your body has achieved.

- Work hard at **ending the comparison game**. (I'm not going to pretend it's easy—most fitness-and-beauty marketing is about getting us to compare and despair.) Still, stop trying to look like someone else, and start trying to look more like yourself! At this age. In your body. As it is right now.

- **Cull, curate, and reframe images of yourself.** Our minds are conditioned to spit out negative messages whenever we see ourselves in the mirror or an unposed photograph. For some reason, we hang on to photos we hate, poring over them as if they held keys to a crime scene! Delete those pics, or acknowledge what's happening—*ep, that's my inner critic pointing out my chicken legs/big belly/under-eye bags.* Then, challenge yourself to come up with one neutral or positive thought: *Damn, I walked all the way up that mountain/Hey, those mountains look like a postcard of Switzerland/I've always loved that sweater.* Extra points if your focus shifts from your appearance to *something outside yourself.*

- **Spring-clean your wardrobe.** How great would it feel to purge the "thin clothes" you've been using to punish yourself with?

- For that matter, stop telling yourself you need to be thin (or fit, or fast, or "healthier") before you can try something new and exciting. Try it now.

- **Thin out your social media feed.** Unfollow any account that drags your body image into the gutter.

- Practice **compliment karma.** Praise one woman without mentioning her appearance. (*Your laugh is contagious!)*

- **Redefine success.** Replace *I'm not thin enough yet* with *what can my body do today that it couldn't a month ago?* Every time you lift, reach, walk, laugh, type, hug, or even nap—that's your body *doing the damn thing.* Celebrate that. Trust that.

You can (and should) use these tools relentlessly, until they become habits. You should come up with your own, and when you do, please share. Make peace with the fact that challenging body image assumptions and talking yourself down from the latest ageist, sizeist, or sexist attack is going to be a daily task. Sort of a household chore. (*Oops, a bunch of outdated messages seem to piling up around here. Guess it's time to take out the trash.)* It's not your fault that you have to keep advocating for yourself—and the fact that the challenges keep coming isn't a comment on your ability to handle your stressors. On the bright side, if enough of us keep taking out this trash, we might actually create a better world for younger women. Wouldn't that feel good?

That said, **the body image monster is sneaky. You haven't seen the last of him/her/it.**

I stopped weighing myself decades ago, but sometimes the monster finds an opening. Deprived of a number on the scale, it can obsess over the size of my clothing or the measurement of my waist. Or just, you know, "fixing myself up." Finding "flattering" clothes, decorating my body to make it fit in better, staring at my wrinkles. For some women, this is a harmless hobby, but for me it's pretty dark. I can see other women going to a similar place with anti-aging serums or laser face treatments or whatever.

That's where I went after a recent hernia surgery. My doctor informed me that I'd need at least two weeks before I could resume exercising, and even then I'd need to begin with light weights and progress slowly. I thought, *Yeah yeah, I'm fit, I can get over it in a week and get back into working out.*

The first days post-surgery were a blur of pain, nausea, and frustration. It was hard to move. What was once strong felt fragile. My scars seemed almost to be talking to me. Slowly, as I lay there, pretty much immobile, I began to fixate on every (perceived) imperfection. Bloating, for starters. My stomach felt completely unfamiliar. I tried to remind myself that this was temporary—and it was—but the body image monster chose that moment to speak. *You'll never get rid of this bloated belly. All your hard-earned muscle will melt away. It's melting already! You'll never be able to lift heavy again. All that strength will be gone. You'll have to start over from scratch.*

I had two choices: I could let these thoughts take over, or I could begin the hard work of prioritizing my mental health and my recovery. The first step was letting go of perfectionism. My body wasn't going to "bounce back," and that was going to have to be okay. Recovery would have to be about listening to what my body needed, one day at a time. It had just gone through trauma, and it deserved kindness. I tried hard to focus on my body's capacity to repair itself, in ways that weren't visible in the mirror.

Full disclosure—I didn't exactly sail through recovery. I had to work hard at it. But eventually, I was able to focus on gentle movements, walking a little more every day with my aging puppy, deep breathing, and the healing power of rest, especially in the form of quality time with my daughter on the couch watching TV.

Resilience, in other words, is our greatest weapon against the body image monster.

Challenge your inner critic

I recently got the chance to do this while looking at a photo of myself, taken in 2022 at Flamenco Beach in Puerto Rico. It's a beautiful scene—pure white sand, tropical vegetation, crashing waves, endless blue sky. But of course my eyes went right to ME, in my bikini, jumping around, having a blast. I skipped right over my big smile and the gorgeous setting. All I could see was the new belly pouch menopause had bestowed upon me. I did all the things: zoomed in, rolled my eyes, and let the body image monster completely out of its box. Finally, I deleted the picture.

Later, I recovered it from my deleted files, not because I had achieved total harmony with my changing body, but because I came to my senses. Why destroy the physical evidence of a wonderful experience? Why go meekly into a tailspin over an innocent belly? Instead, I decided to **talk back to my inner critic.** I went for maximum snark:

Oh, so you don't think my belly should have been exposed to the Puerto Rican public? Shocker! Do you also think I should wear a "less-revealing" swimsuit?

Perhaps a beach burqah? And while we're at it, how about modesty rules for <u>all women, unless they have perfect bodies?</u>

Enforcing it sounds like a bureaucratic nightmare, but you do you!

Exploration: Maria's Inner Critic Counterattack Cue Card

Inciting Incident (Why the Inner Critic Started Yelling):
  Photo of me on the beach

Tactic	Example
Sarcasm and snark	*"Oh, so you don't think my belly should have been exposed to the Puerto Rican public? Shocker! Should I wear a "less-revealing" swimsuit? Perhaps a beach burqah? And while we're at it, how about modesty rules for all women, unless they have perfect bodies?"*
Calm and logic	*And your point is???? Do you think being horrified by my belly will cause it to disappear?*
Refocusing the viewfinder	*"Yeah, yeah, but remember the translucent, aqua waters, found only in Culebra . . . oh, how I miss that beauty. "*
Friendship and forgiveness	*"Aw, you poor, defenseless inner critic. You must feel under attack to get so defensive. I'm sorry you're having to go through this."*
Redirection	*"I hear what you're saying, but can we talk about something different? Preferably something new and different?"*

I encourage you to debate your own inner critic, as often as possible. Give it a try on the next page...

Exploration: The Inner Critic Counterattack Cue Card

Inciting Incident (Why the Inner Critic Started Yelling):

Tactic	Example
Sarcasm and snark	
Calm and logic	
Refocusing the viewfinder	
Friendship and forgiveness	
Redirection	

Exploration: The Charlie Test

When the Body Image monster pops up (and you know it will) get clear on what it's telling you, and ask yourself: Would this be an appropriate message for a happy, self-confident young girl (who just happens to be my daughter)? If not, substitute a better message. Here's an example from a friend:

1. NST (negative self-talk) while looking in the mirror: *Those pants are not flattering. I guess I'm too old to wear tight pants. I need to camouflage my legs.*

2. Run through the Charlie Test. *Would I tell Charlie—or anyone's daughter—any version of what I just told myself? Of course not! I'm not a monster!*

3. CTR (Charlie Test Rewrite): *Never mind how these pants look—the more important issue is that they feel god awful. So uncomfortable. Off to Goodwill with them, I say, after which my closet will have a vacancy. Only comfortably stylish pants need apply.*

Three Step Charlie Test

1. NST: Catch yourself in the middle of negative self-talk.
2. Run through the Charlie Test: (Would I say this to Charlie?)
3. Charlie Test Rewrite: (What would you say instead?)

1. NST (negative self-talk) while looking in the mirror:

2. Run through the Charlie Test. (Would I say this to Charlie or anyone's daughter?)

3. CTR (Charlie Test Rewrite):

Chapter 5: Moving through Menopause

Picture this: It's 2020, at the end of lockdown. I'm standing in front of my gym bag, shoes in hand. I'm exhausted. Not sore, not lazy, but bone-deep tired, as if my joints are encased in concrete. My playlist is ready. I have every reason to go to the gym. But I just stand there, blinking at the wall. This is new for me, and I don't understand it. I mean, I know I don't like it, but beyond that, what?

Why would I, of all people, resist going to the gym to work out? I'd been passionate about moving my body for as long as I could remember. But now, between anxiety, hot flashes, insomnia, and overwhelming fatigue, I seemed to have lost the will to pick up that gym bag.

Everything I just described is a symptom of perimenopause, but it took longer than you'd think to make that connection. For years, I'd stuck with the same formula: 45 minutes on a cardio machine, then 45 minutes of strength training. It was predictable and effective, at least, according to my definition of "effective" at the time. My routine kept me strong, lean, and in control, I thought.

Until one day, it didn't.

But I forced myself to go to the gym and do what I'd always done, hoping to fix the growing fatigue, anxiety, and lack of motivation. But instead of feeling better, I felt worse. Finally, I decided something had to change. I eased off on myself and got curious.

What was holding me back?

What had movement meant to me in the past?

What was changing, and how would I grapple with it?

Did I want to go back to the gym?

If so, how did I want to spend my time there?

Somewhere in all that musing, I rediscovered racquetball, a sport I loved in my teens. It was fast, fierce, fun, and full of people who showed up to compete hard and laugh harder. I couldn't imagine ever stopping, but when I moved to the U.S. I couldn't immediately find a court, and racquetball faded into the background.

But I kept my racquet. And one day, not long after that frozen-gym-bag moment, I picked it up again, got in the car and drove to LA Fitness, excited to join a recreational racquetball league and pick up where I'd left off, obsessing over performance and chasing wins. Racquetball was just as I remembered. It was me who had changed. I played a fun, sweaty set with a friend, but didn't end up joining the league, because I no longer felt that competitive urge. Which was fine! These days I use racquetball to add a sprinkle of spice to my menu of movement. I'll play a couple of times per month.

In a related matter, although I still go to the gym 3 to 4 times a week, I no longer pressure myself to do the same thing each time.

You might be interested to know what other kinds of movement I do.

One recent Tuesday morning, I danced to the Pointer Sister's "I'm So Excited" around the kitchen in my socks, arriving at the stove just in time to flip my daughter's pancake. A few hours later, I spent 45 minutes doing some heavy lifting at the gym, lost in my own world, not making small talk (or even eye contact.) That evening, I walked my three dogs, GG, Luna, and Percy (the oldest and smallest, but undeniably the boss), while listening to Leanne Morgan's "*What in the World?*"

On weekends, you might find me biking on an urban trail, weaving through trees, simply *being* outside.

On vacation, I jump at the chance to hike straight up the hill(and back down).

There's no longer any typical day of movement for me. Where I used to dread any change in my routine, I now see it as a sign of growth and freedom. Instead of a set of plans, goals, and metrics, I rely on something I call the Movement Map. It's big, messy, inspiring, and subject to change.

Now you get to figure this out yourself and design your own Movement Map.

You already know **movement is good for you.** Stronger bones, better heart health, lower risk of disease, sharper mind, happier mood . . . all that is **even better for you** in menopause. Strength training stimulates muscles by exposing them to controlled stress, which forces them to adapt, grow, and get stronger. Impact and weight-bearing activities provide the signal bones need to stay dense and strong. Balance work protects against falls, one of the most significant risks to independence as we age. Exercise increases blood flow, supports neuroplasticity, and improves memory and mood. Regular movement helps manage blood pressure, cholesterol, and insulin sensitivity, three of the key drivers of cardiovascular disease, which becomes the number one health risk for women after menopause.

In short, the role of exercise evolves: before menopause, it keeps you fit; during and after, it becomes the cornerstone of preserving independence and energy in the years ahead.

See what I mean by **good for you?** But you already know that—the basics, at least—and if that were all the motivation you needed, you wouldn't be reading this book and I wouldn't be writing it! As I've said, movement needs to be personalized if it's going to add to your quality of life in a meaningful way. And I promise we'll get into that.

But first, let's go over some basics.

Strength training

If there's one form of movement I'd encourage you to prioritize above all else, it's this. Improved strength is your best defense against everything from bone loss to fatigue. We're not just talking about looking strong. We're talking about *being* strong—physically, mentally, and metabolically.

Strength and resistance training are my personal passions, so I'm always happy when research confirms that what makes me feel good is also good for my health. Better yet, recent research shows that resistance training is particularly beneficial to women in all stages of menopause.
Strength and resistance training:

- Promote bone density

- Strengthen the heart

- Improve mental health

- Help maintain or improve existing muscle

- Increase resting metabolic rate, causing more calories to be burned in a resting state

- Improve focus and cognitive function while reducing depression and anxiety.

If you're new to strength training, don't be intimidated. You don't need to be an expert to get started. Nor do you need barbells or a gym membership. You just need to use resistance—whether that's your own bodyweight, resistance bands, dumbbells, or a heavy laundry basket—to challenge your muscles and help them grow stronger over time. Your first step might be doing squats while holding onto the back of a chair, or push-ups against the kitchen counter. From there, you might progress to a group class, or work with a trainer, or download a plan and take it to a gym—as long as you check in with yourself.

If you don't like the vibe of a workout facility, that's on the facility! Take your business elsewhere. If you don't like working out indoors, check out the many, smaller backyard-and-warehouse-type facilities in most urban areas. You can get stronger without ever touching a piece of gym equipment—through such sports as swimming, martial arts, rock climbing (indoors or out) and many, many more options. If you don't think of yourself as a joiner, feel free to work out alone, or experiment with smaller groups—you never know, these people might become your Fitness Fairies! If you're pressed for time, try for 20-minute sessions. The point is, there's an infinite variety of ways to build strength, so pick one (or several) that fit your personality and preferences.

Myth-busting strength training

- **Lifting weights will make me bulky.** Building noticeable muscle mass actually takes years of intentional training, progressive overload, protein timing, and, most importantly, genetics that most of us don't have. You don't just "accidentally" bulk up. Can we retire this one?

- **Strength training is boring.** Only if you're doing the boring version! So if the thought of "sticking with it for 12 weeks" makes you lose the will, take a breath and try something different.

- **I'm too old to start.** Muscle responds to resistance at any age. Research consistently shows that anyone—in their seventies, eighties, and beyond—can gain strength, build muscle, improve balance, and increase independence.

- **I need to get in shape before I start lifting.** In fact, strength training is *how* you get in shape.

- **Go hard or go home—if you're not sore after lifting, you did it wrong.** Nope. That achy feeling you sometimes get after lifting (known as DOMS , or delayed onset muscle soreness) comes from microscopic tears within muscle fibers. This is normal, temporary stress that signals adaptation, not injury. As your body adjusts to training, soreness usually decreases, even as you continue to get stronger and build muscle.

- **Muscle turns into fat when you stop exercising—and vice versa.**
  Biologically impossible! Muscle and fat are two completely different tissues. One cannot "turn into" the other, just as a strawberry can't turn into a banana. What does happen? Muscle mass may decrease if you stop strength training, and if activity drops but calorie intake stays the same, fat can accumulate.

At first, many of my clients are apprehensive about strength training. But once they realize it can happen anywhere—and take whatever form they prefer—the whole game changes.

Morgan, 61, described herself as "a distance junkie." She ran five, sometimes six, days per week, logging miles as if they were therapy sessions. (In many ways, they were.) Running cleared her mind and gave her structure and stress relief. I met her shortly after she was sidelined by a knee injury. She was feeling pretty miserable.

"I don't know who I am without running," she told me. At first, she rejected the idea of strength training, mainly because it wasn't running! Eventually, through a lot of mindset work, we reframed it: not as a replacement for running, but as a way to rebuild and recover. She started with short, structured sessions: twice a week, for thirty minutes, using dumbbells and her own bodyweight at home. Over time, we increased her sessions to four times per week, 45 to 60 minute sessions, using all the equipment the gym had to offer. She stopped measuring her worth in miles and began to feel strong in new ways. More grounded. More stable. And in much less pain than she'd had in years.

Now she still runs, but less often, and with more intention. "I didn't realize how much I had wrapped my identity around mileage," she says. "Strength training gave me a new way to feel powerful."

Jenny, 49, told me she was doing everything right. Eating clean, getting her steps in, watching her wine intake. But perimenopause had hit hard, and her body was changing in all the predictable ways. She'd picked strength training to tame the belly fat monster—she intended to kick that new fat accumulation to the curb! Doing that would give her back the feeling of control she had relied on for most of her life.

I told Jenny I couldn't promise her fast results, weight loss or fat loss, because that is not something I promise anyone. I did say I could help her get stronger—and begin to notice that her body was capable and deserving of much more than just weight loss. She began a program of progressive resistance training: two full-body sessions per week to start. Within weeks, her sleep improved, her anxiety subsided, and her focus slowly shifted from **how her body looked to what it could do.**

"I came in chasing smaller jeans," she now says. "I stayed because I realized how strong I could be, in my body and in my mind."

In fact, her body composition changed. She did lose fat, some of it from her belly. But that was no longer the point. The goal had shifted from shrinking to owning her space. Now she lifts three times a week. She says it's her anchor, her reset button. Her only regret is not having started sooner.

Cardio

According to the American College of Sports Medicine, "any sport or activity that works large muscle groups, is continually maintained, and performed rhythmically is defined as an aerobic or cardiovascular exercise." In other words, cardio is any movement that strengthens your heart by making it more efficient at delivering oxygen throughout your body. As you increase your aerobic capacity, your heart, lungs, and blood vessels all improve their ability to supply oxygen where it's needed most. This matters even more in midlife, because when estrogen levels drop during menopause, we lose some of its heart-protective effects. That shift can impact cholesterol, blood pressure, and how blood vessels function, raising the risk of heart disease, which is already the number one cause of death for women across all ages.

Please know that that cardio isn't limited to treadmills, spin bikes, or pounding the pavement. If it gets your heart rate up and is sustained over time, it counts. Hiking, swimming, dancing, cycling, cardio kickboxing, many team sports and playing pickleball are all forms of cardiovascular exercise.

Walking, for instance, often gets dismissed as not real exercise, but the research says otherwise. In fact, it's the single most studied and consistently proven form of movement for improving health across the board. Walking reduces the risk of high blood pressure, high cholesterol and diabetes as effectively as running! It's also been linked to improvements in stress, anxiety, and depression. For some of us, walking might be our chance to spend time alone, to clear (or empty) our minds. Perhaps best of all, walking is accessible. You can take a walk just about anywhere, at any pace. So yes, I'm talking about a ten-minute stroll after lunch, a walk-and-talk with a good friend, or a hike on the weekend with a romantic interest. They all count.

My client Angie used to drag herself to the gym for what she described as "boring cardio sessions" on the elliptical and "structured" workouts that took more time than she had. One day, I happened to ask her if she ever hiked in the beautiful mountains behind her house. She did, in fact. Almost every day! "Why punish yourself with boring cardio?" I asked. "You're already doing plenty of it, and in such a gorgeous setting!" It didn't count, Angie answered, because it was fun! For a moment, I was speechless, but once I regained the ability to speak, we worked on reframing. <u>What if the fun movement is actually the best movement?</u> Once Angie started seeing her hikes as valid, the "shoulds" loosened their grip.

Conversations about cardio inevitably center around intensity. You'll hear such terms as Zone 2 training, threshold, VO_2 max, high-intensity interval training (HIIT). If you enjoy nerding out over physiology, go for it, but if all this mystifies you, it's okay. Here's all you really need to know about intensity:

- **Zone 1:** Very light. Easy stroll, chatting effortlessly.

- **Zone 2:** Light to moderate. Brisk walk or gentle cycle. You can talk, but you know you're working.

- **Zone 3:** Moderate to vigorous. Talking gets harder, you'd rather focus on breathing.

- **Zone 4:** Hard. Breathing heavy, sentences are tough.

- **Zone 5:** All-out sprint mode. Only lasts a few seconds.

- **Threshold training (Zone 3-4):** Holding a "comfortably hard" pace (you can talk in short phrases). Great for improving endurance and delaying fatigue.

- **VO$_2$ max workouts (Zone 5):** Short, high-intensity intervals at or near your max effort to boost aerobic capacity, speed, and overall cardiovascular fitness.

  - Think of it as: Threshold keeps you going longer. VO$_2$ max makes you go faster.

- **HIIT (high-intensity interval training)** isn't just "sweat a lot and call it a day." True HIIT means working in short, near-maximal bursts of effort alternated with recovery periods. Classic examples include sprint interval training (SIT) or Tabata protocols (20 sec work/10 sec rest for 8 intervals). Many workouts slapped with a "HIIT" label are really just hard circuits. Good workouts, but not technically HIIT.

- Unless you're training for a race or a specific performance goal, you don't need to track these zones. You don't need to track anything, unless you want to. Some cardio is always better than no cardio. Once you figure that out, you have my permission to tell people you're **in the zone**.

CARDIO POST-IT NOTE

Just move – most days.
Mix up the intensity once in a while.
Do activities you enjoy.
Avoid activities you dread.

It's generally recommended to aim for at least 150-300 minutes of moderate-intensity cardio or 75-150 minutes of high-intensity cardio per week. You don't have to do it all in long sessions—intervals as short as ten minutes add up over time.

Here are a few options to consider:

- **Jogging and running,** the way you did as a kid, with no destination in mind.

- **Jogging and running, the grown-up way**—perhaps a group run, track workouts, races.

- **Aerobic or cardio-dance classes, Zumba, Jazzercise,** and the many local variations of dancing like no one's watching. If you like this kind of thing, you'll be having so much fun you won't even notice how sweaty you're getting or how hard your heart is working.

- **Swimming and aqua aerobics** are excellent low-impact exercise options that absolutely build cardio capacity.

- **Cycling,** indoors or out.

- **Racquet sport, from racquetball to tennis to squash to pickleball.**

- **Team sports, from soccer to kickball to Ultimate.**

- **Ice- or roller-skating. Hiking, trekking or rucking,** also known as hiking with a weighted pack.

Linda hadn't been on a bike in decades, but during the pandemic she dusted off her old cruiser and started riding around the neighborhood for ten minutes now and then. She soon graduated to 15–20 mile weekend rides. Now, she considers cycling her "therapy on two wheels."

After years of putting everyone else first, Carla was desperate for "me time." I knew she loved music, so I suggested she try a beginner's cardio dance class. At first, she felt a little embarrassed by the choreography, but the energy and music quickly won her over. The class became her weekly escape, her time to move, laugh, shake off stress, and be in the moment.

Myth-busting cardio

- **Running is the "best" form of cardio.** If you enjoy running, it's the best. If you don't, it's not! The best cardio is the one you'll actually do.

- **Unless you're over a certain age—then running is bad for you, and you should stop doing it, even if you love it.** You may have to adjust your distances, speed or rest schedule, but you absolutely do not have to stop running!

- **Cardio only counts if you do it for 60 minutes straight.** Not true—research shows that even short bouts, 10 or 15 minutes at a time, add up and provide the same health benefits as longer sessions.

- **Fasted cardio** (working out on an empty stomach) **burns more fat.** I mean . . . maybe a little more fat? But not enough to make a statistical difference.

- **Zone 2 cardio is the best for fat loss.** It is effective for sustainable fat loss and metabolic health, but it's only] "the best" if it's the only type you'll do. HIIT or other well-designed protocols are also effective for weight loss and the most important thing to remember is that individual preference and consistency are key.

Flexibility, mobility, and balance

I have to admit I spent decades avoiding what I thought of as "stretching," because it didn't sound fun. But as I get older—and as I lose count of the injuries I've sustained—I've incorporated flexibility and mobility into my routine. I begin each workout with a five-minute mobility sequence of four basic exercises. Repeating the same moves keeps things simple and efficient. The purpose is to prepare my body for movement, not to design something new each time. That's what I do, and you're welcome to give it a try. Most important is that you figure out what works for you. For instance, you might be more drawn to a gentle yoga routine in a group or just adapting a few poses into your daily routine.

Flexibility and mobility are important not only for recovery and improved performance, but also for preventing injuries and improving posture. Although often used interchangeably, flexibility and mobility are two different things.

Flexibility is the amount your soft tissue (muscle, tendons, ligaments) can lengthen—how far you can bend toward your toes before your hamstrings stop you, for instance. This becomes especially important in midlife because soft tissues gradually lose elasticity with age, which can limit range of motion and increase susceptibility to strains or joint pain. Add hormonal changes into the mix, like lower estrogen, which affects collagen and connective tissue and flexibility work becomes less about doing the splits and more about keeping joints moving comfortably, preventing pain, supporting joint health, and maintaining functional movement.

Mobility is the ability of a joint to move actively through a range of motion—how far a golfer's hips move through a swing, for instance, or the length of a sprinter's stride. Different physical activities require different ranges of motion, but in general, there's no reason not to maintain or improve your range of motion. Improving range of motion in midlife is essential for staying mobile, independent, and active. It helps protect joints, ease muscle tension, and lower the risk of injury and makes everyday movements, like walking, reaching, bending, and even getting up from the floor, easier and more comfortable. In short, better range of motion means better quality of life.

One of my clients, Lena, loved gardening, but squatting down to pull weeds left her knees aching for days. She thought she'd have to give up the hobby she loved but once she started improving her range of motion with hip and ankle mobility drills, gardening stopped feeling like punishment for her joints. She could crouch down, reach forward, and stand back up smoothly, getting back the joy of doing what she loved outdoors.

Robin discovered ashtanga yoga, by accident, at a snowboarding camp thirty years ago. She was surprised at how challenging-and-yet-calming it was, but with all the long-distance running and cycling she was doing, she didn't see how she could make time for what she thought of as stretching. By the time she started working with me, she'd been injured often enough to start really listening to her body. She still cycles, but shorter distances, and she doesn't run, but she's always practicing one kind of yoga or another. "I've never gotten the message that yoga is something you age out of," she says, "and as I get older I want more flexibility, not less. There's always something new to learn in yoga. It's not something you achieve, it's something you practice."

There are three main ways to improve both flexibility and mobility:

- **Dynamic stretching,** also known as range-of-motion exercise, is designed to prepare the body for what it's about to do in the "main event"—slowly kicking your leg through every phase of your running stride, for instance. It is generally the top choice for preparing the body for movement and enhancing performance (e.g., jump height, muscle strength, coordination) and is recommended as part of a warm-up before exercise. It increases blood flow, prepares the body for movement, and has a positive effect on power and speed. Research indicates that 5 minutes of repeated movements, or 30–60 seconds per movement, is beneficial for flexibility and mobility before activity.

- **Static stretching** (holding a stretch for 15–30 seconds) is best as a cooldown tool after exercise. It can increase range of motion and flexibility. However, static stretching before exercise has *not* been shown to prevent injuries and may even increase injury risk when done before strength training. Also, there is evidence that static stretching can temporarily reduce muscle strength and power if performed immediately before high-intensity activity, making it a better choice for post-exercise and cooldowns rather than the start of a workout. Research indicates that 2–4 sets of 10–30 seconds per muscle group is sufficient to improve flexibility. For long-term flexibility improvements, stretching for four or more minutes per muscle five times a week is recommended.

- **Myofascial release** (through massage or foam rolling) is particularly effective for recovery or improving flexibility with minimal risk of performance impairment and can be used both before and after exercise. It is strongly associated with post-exercise recovery, reducing soreness and fatigue, and providing non-pharmacological support for chronic pain and tension. Unlike static stretching, MFR is less likely to impair muscle power and may modestly improve strength and performance if used in a warm-up or recovery routine.

Each modality serves its own purpose. A mix of all three tends to offer the most benefit.

Ideally, make time for stretching and flexibility two to three times per week, as well as before and after workouts. But, as always, take this recommendation and make it work for you. If stretching bores you, try for 5 minutes most days.

Balance is integral to fitness, but often overlooked, especially before age catches up with us. (It's hard to care about "fall prevention" when you're twenty!) But because the risk of osteoporosis increases exponentially during menopause, it's important to work on maintaining your ability to, for example, stand on one leg, hold yourself upright, or walk through a dark room without tripping on a sleeping dog. (Yes, it's much harder to balance when you can't see or when you're wearing noise-canceling headphones.) The good news is that you have the power to maintain balance almost indefinitely. You can learn a new balance-based discipline, such as Tai Chi, or simply challenge your balance during daily activities. Try balancing on one leg while brushing your teeth, doing dishes, or reaching for something. Once that becomes easy, try moving the nonstanding leg around to challenge your balance even more (little circles, up and down). I love to include unilateral exercises in my strength training—try doing standing shoulder presses on one leg or a side lunge hop to a full, single-leg stop. This last one builds balance and power and adds high-impact for your bones. In general, almost anything you can do on two legs is more challenging on one.

Yoga and Tai Chi are two forms of movement that truly stand the test of time. We can all picture groups of older adults flowing through Tai Chi in the park, reminding us that movement doesn't have to be punishing and doesn't have to stop as we age. At its core, yoga is smart movement that blends balance, flexibility, and mobility, all of which are especially valuable in midlife. And the benefits go beyond just feeling limber. Research shows that yoga can reduce stress, improve sleep, and even ease some of the physical and urogenital symptoms that come with menopause. What's encouraging is that the improvements don't require a massive time investment; just a couple of sessions a week for about ten weeks can make a real difference in well being and quality of life.

Sometimes called "meditation in motion," **Tai Chi** feels like moving through water in slow motion. It's a practice of flowing, low-impact movements that blend flexibility, balance, and mindfulness all in one. The beauty of Tai Chi is that it's gentle on the joints yet surprisingly powerful for stability. Research consistently shows that regular Tai Chi practice helps reduce the risk of falls, improves balance and mobility, and even boosts mood and sleep. The best part is that you don't need fancy gear or a gym membership. A living room, backyard, or a quiet corner of the park will do. With its slow, deliberate transitions and focus on posture and breath, Tai Chi builds flexibility without deep stretches and steadiness without strain. It's also a perfect midlife movement because it brings together what so many of us are looking for: calm, connection, and confidence in our bodies.

Hybrid workout

Hybrid workouts aren't just "one thing." They mix and match cardio, flexibility, and strength training, as well as build strength, endurance, mobility, balance, mental grit, and even social connection—sometimes all at once.

Here are some great examples—and new ones are being invented all the time.

Rock climbing: Every climb is different, so your body and brain adapt in real time. Indoors or outdoors, rock climbing is an intuitive blend of strength, cardio, flexibility, grip, mental focus, and adventure. One of the best parts? The climbing world is famously close-knit, so you're not just building strength—you're building friendships.

Cardio kickboxing: A workout that combines explosive cardio with rotational strength and coordination. It's high-intensity but also skill-based, combining rhythm, balance, and agility while delivering a powerful conditioning workout.

A **via ferrata** is a protected type of climbing that combines hiking with iron rungs, ladders, and cables fixed to the rock. Many were first built in the Italian Alps during World War I to move troops through the mountains. I tried it recently and found it exhilarating, as well as the scariest thing I've ever done. I would most definitely do it again. This is the epitome of a hybrid workout: climbing ladders bolted into cliffs, traversing narrow ledges, gripping cables, all while hiking in between. It's functional fitness in the most adventurous setting possible.

Rowing (on water or erg): A seamless combination of cardio and strength, engaging legs, back, core, and arms in one fluid, rhythmic motion. Rowing is low-impact yet high-return, building both stamina and muscular endurance. Indoor and outdoor rowing share the same full-body cardio and strength benefits, but rowing on the water adds extra layers. The boat rocks (literally), so your core and balance get a surprise challenge, and changes in wind, current, and scenery keep things fresh.

Martial arts: Full-body strength, balance, strategy, mindfulness, flexibility, and even philosophy. These practices are as much mental as they are physical, keeping both body and brain sharp.

Pilates: Precision, control, and core strength meet mobility and posture training. Pilates builds deep stabilizing muscles, improves alignment, and teaches body awareness, making every other form of movement (from lifting to hiking) safer and more efficient.

Honorable mention: Blue Zones

Blue Zones are specific regions in the world where people consistently live longer, healthier lives, often reaching the age of 100 at rates significantly higher than the average population. Researchers have identified five main Blue Zones in Japan, Sardinia, Greece, Costa Rica, and southern California. These farflung places have a few notable things in common, including diet (mostly plant-based, unprocessed, fish/poultry vs red meat, minimal added sugars), natural movement, social connections, a sense of community and purpose, and moderate alcohol consumption. We'll focus more on the other aspects in later chapters, but when it comes to movement, Blue Zones flip the idea of *exercise* on its head. In Blue Zones, movement isn't a class, a time slot, or a chore. It's woven into the fabric of daily life.

People in Blue Zones don't struggle to get their steps in. They walk to visit friends, strength-train their bodies as they tend their gardens and haul firewood, raise their heart rates by herding animals up and down mountains and maintain strength, flexibility and joy by dancing at frequent communal celebrations. Note that none of these activities are done to burn fat or "earn" meals! In Blue Zones,

- Mobility and flexibility don't automatically decline with age. In Okinawa, it's common to sit on the floor, which means standing up and sitting down multiple times a day. That's a natural way to maintain hip mobility, balance, and leg strength well into old age.

- Movement becomes social glue. Dancing, walking to neighbors' homes, cooking or fishing or building rock walls together—all of this movement fosters connection. In fact, much of this movement is done *in* connection, with friends and family of all generations.

- They're not chasing personal records. They're chasing life. Consistency over intensity. Blue Zone movement proves that the human body is designed to thrive when activity is consistent, joyful, and functional.

High impact and weightbearing: why they matter

Both these types of movement play an important role in **bone health**, as I'm about to explain. But first, what are they?

High-impact refers to movements that generate a forceful impact on the bones—any activity in which both feet leave the ground at the same, creating a jolt through the body when it returns to earth. Think hopping, skipping, jumping, or sprinting. Think jogging, cardio dance, circuit training that includes intervals of jumping, or even jumping into puddles after it rains, because why not?

By **weight-bearing,** I mean any activity that requires your body to work against gravity, exerting a gravitational force on the skeleton. This includes such activities as walking, hiking, climbing stairs, or performing weighted exercises such as lunges and squats.

Without getting too sciency, here's why weight-bearing exercises, such as resistance training and high-impact exercise, are so good for your bones: every time you lift, push, or pull, your muscles tug on your bones while gravity adds extra force. That tug creates little stress signals in your skeleton, and your bone's "smart sensors" (called osteocytes) pick up on it, telling the bone-building crew (osteoblasts) to get to work and reminding the demolition crew (osteoclasts) to chill out. The result? Stronger and denser bones.

Weight-bearing and high-impact movements often overlap, making it easy to integrate both into a single workout or daily activities. For example,

- Hiking uphill with a backpack is a weightbearing activity. Hopping over rocks or puddles adds moments of high-impact.

- Squatting to pull weeds in your garden loads your muscles and bones; jumping up to a standing position adds impact.

- Adding a hop at the top of a step-up circuit at the gym combines weightbearing and high impact.

- Walking lunges load your bones nicely—turn a few into jumping lunges to add impact.

What does this have to do with bones?

Both **high-impact** and **weightbearing** activities can help maintain **bone density**.

While our bones stop growing in length in our early twenties, they can still increase in thickness and strength throughout life. That process does tend to slow down during menopause, since estrogen plays a key role in maintaining bone density. Subjecting your bones to the mechanical stress of weight-bearing and high-impact exercise helps mitigate the risk of bone loss and osteoporosis by stimulating new bone growth and maintaining the bone density you already have. Research shows that high-impact movement can have a significant benefit in helping your skeleton become denser and stronger over time.

A word of caution

If you've been diagnosed with **osteoporosis**, you'll need to weigh the benefits of high-impact activities against the increased risk of bone fractures. "Let's-jump-off-the-biggest-box" or plyometric drills may not be the safest choice, especially if you've had spinal fractures, multiple breaks, or a history of falls. But that doesn't mean you're stuck in bubble wrap. Lower-to-moderate-impact options like step-ups, or even smaller hops can still challenge your bones in a safe way and you can still load your bones safely with resistance training. The key is to tailor it to your situation and, ideally, check in with your healthcare provider or fitness professional before you jump—literally—into something new.

If you've been diagnosed with **osteopenia**, there are generally no restrictions. In fact, any type of high-impact activities can help slow down—or even stop—the progression to osteoporosis.

What if you have **arthritis**? What about **injuries you never completely recovered from**—that limit your mobility or strength? First of all, welcome to the club! Few of us make it to midlife without a few dings and limitations, especially if we've led active lives. Second, please know that **avoiding injury doesn't have to mean avoiding movement itself.** You may have been told to "avoid overloading joints." It's a good idea, but that can mean a lot of things and it's important to adjust your movement depending on what injuries or degenerative conditions you're dealing with.

For example, the hip and neck injuries I sustained while in the military prohibit me from doing a lot of forms of higher-impact or repetitive motion workouts. I used to do a lot of box jumps as part of my high-intensity training, but that no longer feels good to my neck or hips, so I swapped it out for a combo of heavy leg presses and ball slams. I still get some of that intensity but none of the jarring impact. To be honest, I was bored at first, but now I can't imagine doing it any other way. My body feels so much stronger, and that's addictive in the best way. I still make sure to include moderate-impact fun to show my bones some love: jump squats, skaters, or mini hops on the BOSU, because variety keeps me sane.

One client of mine had been in an internal battle over not being able to run anymore due to her arthritic knees—she'd always run. It kept her sane, she said. Without it, she felt a bit lost. She laughed when I first suggested water aqua jogging, but when I offered to check out a class with her, she agreed to try it—once. (I figured my own achy skeleton could use a break from gravity.) After the class, she had to admit that not only had she felt zero pain, she'd had maximum fun!

Another client who'd been scared into immobility by a diagnosis of osteoporosis in her spine began a program of progressive resistance training, with a focus on spinal stability. She's thriving.

Yet another client tried all the conservative treatments before agreeing to knee replacement surgery. When her doctor tried to discourage her from a long-planned European bike trip post-surgery, she pushed back. Eventually, they compromised—she biked from Switzerland into France by e-bike, giving her new joint a chance to acclimate, while still bearing weight, breathing hard, and embracing movement and adventure.

Can menopausal hormone therapy (MHT) help me build bone density and/or slow bone loss?

I get this question a lot. Extensive peer-reviewed research shows that MHT is associated with improvements in bone mineral density and a reduced risk of fractures in postmenopausal women. Research also shows that exercise, particularly resistance and high-impact training, promotes new bone formation and strength. Not surprisingly, combining both exercise and MHT is more effective than either strategy on its own.

That said, I'll stay in my lane. Recommending (or discouraging) MHT is outside my scope of practice and expertise. It's a highly individual decision. My goal is simply to share the science in plain language, so you can have informed conversations with your doctor about what's best for you.

Nuts and bolts

How often should you work out? What kind of intensity? Should you join a gym?

The short answer: it depends. As always, showing up regularly matters more than how hard you go on any single day. Ideally, your Movement Map will include a very personalized mix of cardio, strength, flexibility, and balance—and we'll start designing that soon. Every woman's body, history, and preferences are different, but research does give us solid sweet spots to aim for. Think of the following as general guidelines, and remember that I don't expect you to do *all* these things, *all* the time!

- **Strength training:** 2 to 3 sessions per week. Aim for 6–8 sets per muscle group per week, using a weight that pushes you to fatigue in the 8–12 rep range. RT is your best tool for muscle, bone density, and metabolic health.

- **Balance:** 2–3 times per week, either on its own or folded into strength training. Personally, I love incorporating unilateral moves (such as single-leg deadlifts) and exercises that shift my center of gravity to challenge balance and coordination, without adding extra time to my workouts.

- **Cardio:** Approximately 150 minutes of moderate-intensity cardio activities per week.

- **High impact:** 2 to 3 times a week. As with balance work, this can be incorporated into your strength training workouts.

- **HIIT:** 2–3 times per week, with 6–8 short bursts (20–30 seconds) of high effort followed by 1–3 minutes of recovery. I like to finish some of my workouts on a bike or treadmill with a few minutes of HIIT. That way it doesn't take an extra day. Efficiency is my jam.

- **Flexibility and mobility:** Try to do this on most days, either as a short standalone session or tacked on to the end of your workouts. Even 1 minute in between Zoom calls counts. I like to keep it simple with mobility flows (think hip circles, shoulder rolls, cat-cows) and stretches that target the areas I use most, so it feels doable and keeps me moving smoothly.

Real life isn't a lab

The guidelines I just shared come from research and research is about averages, not about *you*. One person's Orange Theory is another person's personal visit to hell, and that's perfectly fine. Some women thrive on several short walks scattered through the day, while others alternate seasons of training with periods of recovery. Maybe you play tennis in the summer and swim in the winter, or switch between hiking and dance classes depending on your mood. Think of movement less like a lifelong marriage and more like speed-dating—you can try different things, enjoy them while they last, and move on when you're ready for a change.

But is it enough? Boy, is this a familiar anxiety! Some of us have had this worry in one form or another for as long as we can remember. Social media influencers and fitness gurus perpetuate this fear by promoting extreme workouts that promise rapid results. For women in midlife, this message comes with an extra dose of ageism—not only should we do *more*, lose *more* fat and gain *more* muscle, we should also engage in a pointless battle with wrinkles and, ultimately, mortality!

You have my permission to ignore these destructive messages. A Movement Map is about the journey, not the stats. The real question is: *What kind of movement gives you the biggest bang for your buck in midlife?* What's backed by research, and what's worth doing when time and energy are in short supply? Finally—and this is **not** optional—what's fun/challenging/adventuresome/soothing enough to keep you interested?

Rest and recovery

They sound simple, but . . . not really. If you grew up participating in competitive sports—during the no-pain/no-gain era—you might have gotten the idea that you can rest when you're injured (or old). And then, as an adult, you've been told that if you "listen to your body" it will tell you when to rest. But . . . how do we do that, exactly?

Here's the thing—your body needs time to repair itself. That process of repair makes it stronger. That means at least one true rest day after demanding workouts as well as embracing active recovery, by which I mean easy movements such as walking, easy bike rides, restorative yoga, stretching, or meditation.

And let's be clear: recovery doesn't have to be complicated. There's a whole industry selling cold plunges, compression sleeves, and other supposedly essential recovery tools. Sure, some of these extras can feel refreshing and enjoyable, but they're not necessary.

Chapter 6: Design Your Movement Map

Now that you know what to do, get out your calendar, pen in the recommended amounts and types of movement, and remember: LIVE, LAUGH, LOVE.

Just kidding. Let's make a plan that actually works. Actually, a map. The kind of map you'd want to guide you through an extended journey (not a bad way to look at menopause) or even the rest of your life, as opposed to a prefab map that shows you **one route** and tells you to **stick to it.** Because what if you hit an obstacle? What if your plan—or your mood—changes? After all, there may be days when adventure matters more to you than core strength, and visa versa. In other words, an editable, adaptable, expandable map.

I'll be your guide, but you're the mapmaker. To get there, you'll need to look back at where you've been. Let's start there.

Exploration: Looking Back

Get out your kit. Below, list all the movement/fitness/exercise/sports activities you've tried. Include fitness classes, weight workouts at home or the gym, walking, hiking, running, cycling, team sports, yoga, pilates, etc. It doesn't matter if you only tried something once or if you last did it 30 years ago. Use whatever shorthand makes sense to you. Include anything that seems significant to you. (And of course, feel free to exclude anything that doesn't.)

Activity	Notes
Walking after school	
That hot yoga class (once)	
Couch to 5k (Jan-Mar)	

Maria's Good, Should–and more!

Grab a colored pencil or pen and review your Looking Back list on the last page.

- Put a big star (preferably in your favorite color) next to anything that feels (or felt) GOOD.
- Put an X next to anything that feels (or felt) SHOULD.
- Some entries might sit there without either an X or a star. Some might have both.
- **Transfer anything you marked with a star to the chart on the next page**.
- Here's my example:

Activity	Notes
Cardio Dance ☆	*I love that cardio dance class so much! I look forward to it all week!*
Lower-your-blood-pressure program my doctor "strongly suggested" I do ✗	*I hated it. I had to wear a step-counter and got a report card at the end of every week. It sucked all the joy out of taking a walk and I felt like a kid being shamed for a bad report card.*
Couch to 5K ☆ ✗	*I started running to manage my weight, and it worked, which was nice, but it turned out I also loved to run, which was even better. I'm still running, but because of injuries, I run longer distances fewer days per week. Meanwhile, though my weight hasn't changed, my waist has grown three inches. I still love the physical feeling of running, but I struggle with thinking that if I went back to my old running routine, I would lose this belly, which is something I should want to accomplish. On the other hand, I could get injured by going back to my old routine, and staying injury free while still enjoying running is good. So is running both a good and a should for me?*

Exploration: Good, Should—and more!

Grab a colored pencil or pen and review your **Looking Back** list on the last page.
- Put a big star (preferably in your favorite color) next to anything that feels (or felt) GOOD.
- Put an X next to anything that feels (or felt) SHOULD.
- Some entries might sit there without either an X or a star. Some might have both.
- Transfer anything you marked with a star to the chart below.

Activity	Notes

Exploration: Clean out the Fridge

If you've spent years forcing your body to move in ways that felt punishing or performative, or if you've been chasing an ideal that never seems to arrive, this process may be harder than you think. It's not just about finding new workouts; it's about unlearning the old rules. That takes guts. Put on some rubber gloves, because I have a feeling you're going to drag some oooooooold ideas about fitness out of that ice box.

- The no pain/no gain meatloaf you tell yourself you're about to reheat, even though it won't taste any better than it did thirty years ago.
- The real-women-don't-sweat frozen dinner with few calories and even less flavor.
- The new year/new you bottled salsa that's lost every bit of flavor—at this point, is it even safe for human consumption?

What old beliefs or rules about movement can you throw in the trash? Include anything that feels outdated, unhelpful, or downright harmful. Anything that "worked" once but no longer does, no matter how hard you try to start over. Take your time. Remember, you learned these messages over many years and from many sources, and some of them are sneaky.

- *I have to take reformer classes, because I heard that's how you get "long and lean." But A: I can't afford them. And B: A long-and-lean lie detector in the back of my mind is going off.*
- *I was in such good shape ___ years ago when I played varsity _____. If I can't get my old body back, what's the point?*

Now it's your turn. What are you ready to throw the hell out?**:**

Okay, now that you've made some room in the fridge, what sounds good?

We'll draft this map by using the insights you've gained so far to yield multiple possibilities for movement, in your daily life and in your wildest dreams. Ideally, you'll come up with ways to fit strength, cardio, balance, flexibility—and much more—into a typical week, or an anything-but-typical year.

On the following pages, you'll see three different templates. You'll get a chance to pick one, or come up with your own. Whatever you decide, your map should include these three areas:

Neighborhood

This is the place for ride-or-die movement activities—things you already do, or would like to do, on a semi-regular basis. Running with friends, commuting to work by foot or bike, working out, or taking classes at a convenient gym—all those belong in your neighborhood. If you tried morning hatha yoga on a recent vacation and thought, "I like the way this makes me feel—I'd like to do this regularly, in real life," that activity goes in your neighborhood. (Yes, even if you haven't started yet or figured out the specifics.) In a perfect world, your neighborhood is full of movement that doesn't require a lot of planning or scheduling and takes anywhere from ten minutes to an hour or so. Note: "Neighborhood" is a way of thinking rather than a specific place. It means comfortable, familiar, habitual, and it fits into the flow of your day.

Outings

Located just outside your Neighborhood, Outings add a little spice, a way to mix things up. This is where you'd put a series of weekend hikes, taking a one-time pickleball or pilates class—maybe they'll end up in your Neighborhood?—or driving across town to move your body in a way that takes a little extra planning.

Adventures

Adventures are set aside from real life. They can take place on vacation or serve as the main reason for the vacation. Adventures include expeditions that take you out of your regular routine—walking ten miles a day while exploring a new city or spending a week learning to surf or scuba-dive or gravel-bike or slackline. My clients have signed up for month-long challenges that involve checking out every local hike or bike trail in their home towns and meeting new friends while they do it.

Exploration: Movement Map Brainstorming

Generate a list of possible activities for the three areas of your map. Revisit Looking Back explorations for ideas. Don't worry about logistics or scheduling just yet—the point is to spit out a lot of ideas. An eraser and colored pencils will be helpful here.

Activity	Neighborhood, Outing, or Adventure	Strength, Cardio, Mobility, Hybrid, Blue Zone	Time: how long you want to spend doing this
Tennis	*Neighborhood*	*Hybrid?*	*60 min, 3 x a week*
Lifting with trainer	*Neighborhood*	*Strength*	*60 min, 2 x a week*
Swimming with dolphins	*Adventure*	*Hybrid?*	*4 days in Key West*
Helping build a garden at the school	*Outing*	*Blue Zone*	*Every Sunday for a month*

Here's some more space to brainstorm!

Activity	Neighborhood, Outing, or Adventure	Strength, Cardio, Mobility, Hybrid, Blue Zone	Time: how long you want to spend doing this

But wait—there's **more!**

- What feels accessible or enjoyable right now, even if it's not what you used to do? For now, don't worry about logistics, just add it to the list.

- What are you hoping to feel more of these days? Energy, strength, ease, connection? Think about types of movement that might promote those good feelings. Again, don't stress out over the details, just add to the list.

- Is there anything you're curious about trying, even if you're not sure you'll like it? Add it.

- Include some Blue Zone activities—gardening, construction, dancing at weddings—surely you can think of other examples from your life. Lifting toddlers? Building a rock wall or patio? Kayaking across a lake to get to a birthday party? Volunteering building trails at a park?

Start mapping!

In the next few pages, you'll see three different styles of maps, followed by a few pages of icons that represent different kinds of movement. Choose a template, grab some scissors and cut out a bunch of icons (more than you think you'll need). The idea is to experiment with different arrangements on your map. You can move the icons around between regions. Your map can represent a week, a month or a year of your life—whatever makes the most sense to you.

You liked the yoga retreat so much you decided to get certified as a teacher. Your adventure just moved into your neighborhood.

Remember—your movement map is a work in progress. I encourage you to start playing around with it. Make a mess. See what a week of movement might look like. Every time you create a pleasing arrangement, take a picture of it. That way, you'll soon have a library of possible movement scenarios. And then, just follow your map and see what happens. Make notes about what worked, what didn't, and what new ideas you've had.

In the next chapter, we'll talk about the motivation required to take your movement map to the next level.

Here's what my map looked like in the early stages: At first, I gravitated toward words and actions.

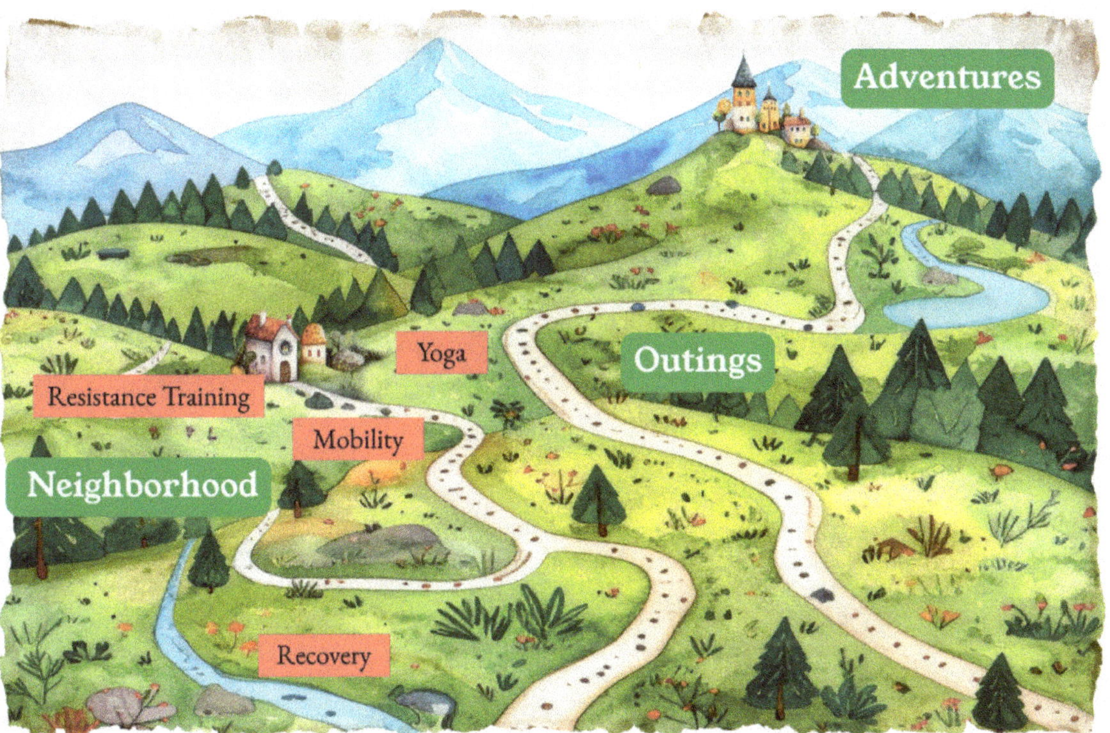

Later, as I started having some real fun with it, I moved to adding only icons because they are more flexible in interpretation and let me visualize different things depending on how I look at them. I included in my Neighborhood activities that I plan on doing regularly at least a few times per week. My Outings are occasional weekends or events in my community, and my Adventures are all about filling my cup: recovery, going back to my roots, and exploration. To me, this represents joy!

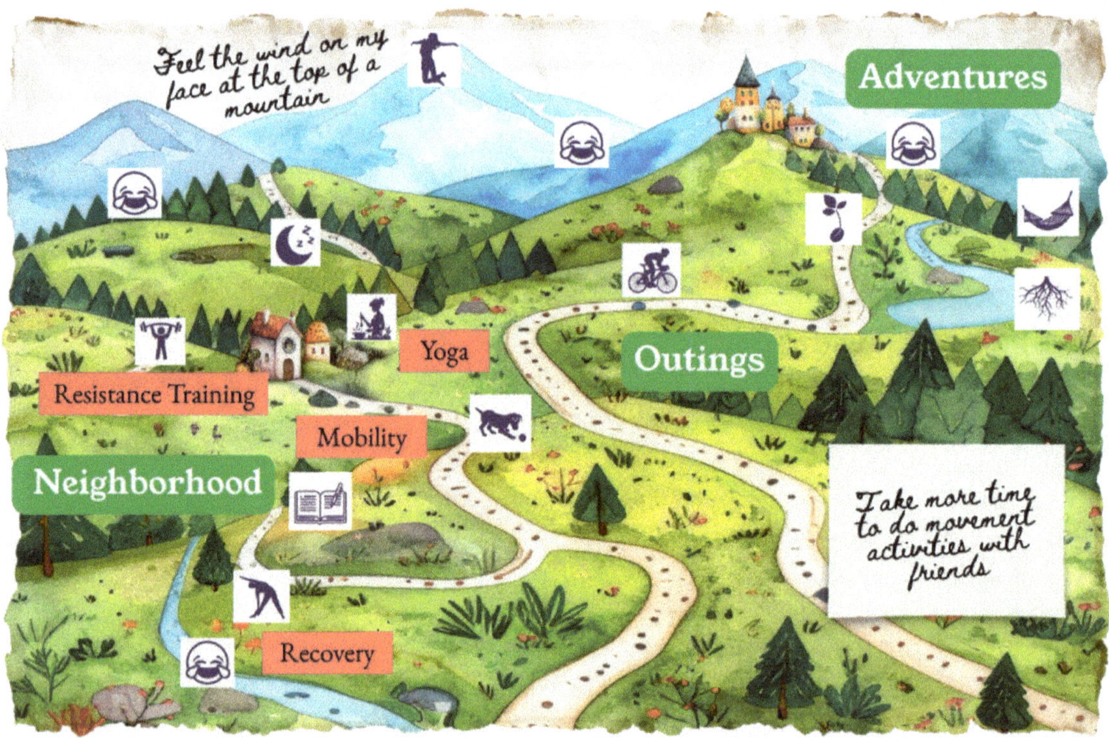

My map is covered with notes, written in pencil, of course, because erasability = flexibility! Eventually, you could tape or glue the icons into a more permanent form. Or take pictures of several different arrangements.

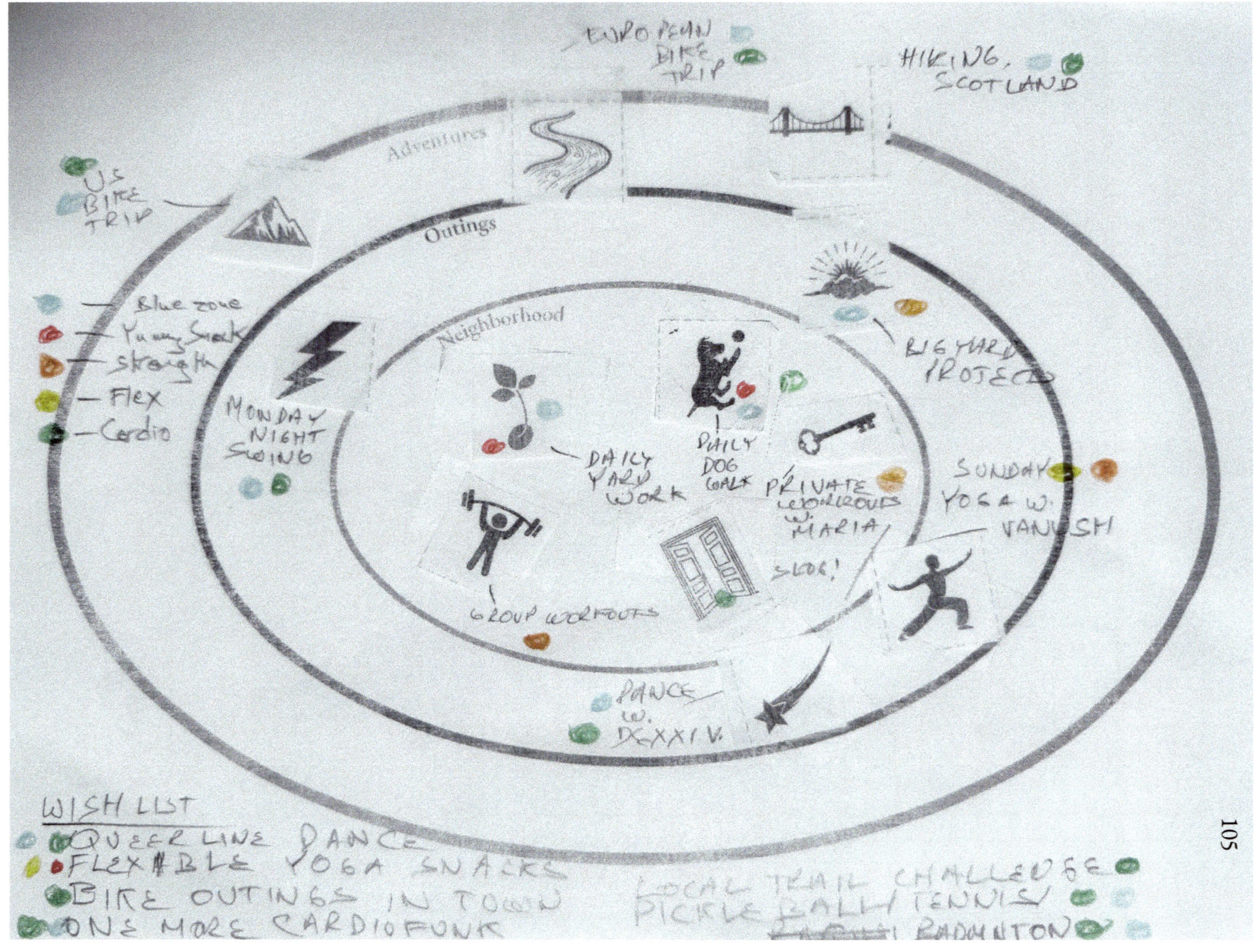

EUROPEAN BIKE TRIP
HIKING, SCOTLAND
US BIKE TRIP
Adventures
Outings
Neighborhood
Blue zone
Yummy Snack
Strength
Flex
Cardio
MONDAY NIGHT SWING
DAILY YARD WORK
DAILY DOG WALK
BIG YARD PROJECT
PRIVATE WORKOUTS W. MARIA
SLEEP!
GROUP WORKOUTS
SUNDAY YOGA W. VANLSH
DANCE W. DCXXIV.
WISH LIST
QUEER LINE DANCE
FLEX#BLE YOGA SNACKS
BIKE OUTINGS IN TOWN
ONE MORE CARDIOFUNK
LOCAL TRAIL CHALLENGE
PICKLE BALL/TENNIS
BADMINTON

Adventures

Trip to Spain to learn flamenco

More fun!

Neighborhood

Movement Snack

Resistance Training

Gentle Movement

5K

Movement Snack

One Small Step

More fun!

Outings

Join a league

Maybe I can find nature walk or hiking group

Build Your Own

The following pages contain cut-outs and symbols/ Movement Snack icons that you can cut out and use on your own maps. If you'd prefer not to cut up this book–or if you want extra copies–you can download PDFs of these templates online by scanning the QR code below or by visiting newmovesinmenopause.com

Move & Play

Wander	5k	Something New	Zumba	Flexibility	Cardio
Boxing	5k	Something New	Bicycling	Flexibility	Cardio
Hiking	10k	Joyful Movement	Bicycling	Marathon	Cardio
Jumping	10k	Joyful Movement	Hike	Rebound	Cardio
Repel	HIIT	Gentle Movement	Hike	Skip Hop	Gardening
Swim	HIIT	One Small Step	Strength	Pickleball	Gardening
Swim	Jog	Power Walk	Strength	Pole Dance	Skydiving
Swim	Jog	Yoga In The Park	Strength	Balance	Spinning
Sprint	Barre	Resistance Training	Strength	Aqua Jogging	Tennis
Tai Chi	Play	Resistance Training	Strength	Stair Climbing	Aerobics
Carpool	Play	Resistance Training	Rowing	Basketball	Aerobics
Yoga	Play	Play With Pets	Recovery	Water Aerobics	Mobility
Pilates	Walk	Play With Pets	Recovery	Table Tennis	Mobility
Sprint	Walk	Movement Snack	Recovery	Racquetball	Mobility
Climb	Walk	Movement Snack	Recovery	Martial Arts	Just Move
Dance	Run	Movement Snack	Recovery	Group Exercise	Just Move
Dance	Run	Movement Snack	Recovery	Group Exercise	Just Move
Dance	Run	Movement Snack	Recovery	Group Exercise	Just Move

Move & Play

Wander	5k	Something New	Zumba	Flexibility	Cardio
Boxing	5k	Something New	Bicycling	Flexibility	Cardio
Hiking	10k	Joyful Movement	Bicycling	Marathon	Cardio
Jumping	10k	Joyful Movement	Hike	Rebound	Cardio
Repel	HIIT	Gentle Movement	Hike	Skip Hop	Gardening
Swim	HIIT	One Small Step	Strength	Pickleball	Gardening
Swim	Jog	Power Walk	Strength	Pole Dance	Skydiving
Swim	Jog	Yoga In The Park	Strength	Balance	Spinning
Sprint	Barre	Resistance Training	Strength	Aqua Jogging	Tennis
Tai Chi	Play	Resistance Training	Strength	Stair Climbing	Aerobics
Carpool	Play	Resistance Training	Rowing	Basketball	Aerobics
Yoga	Play	Play With Pets	Recovery	Water Aerobics	Mobility
Pilates	Walk	Play With Pets	Recovery	Table Tennis	Mobility
Sprint	Walk	Movement Snack	Recovery	Racquetball	Mobility
Climb	Walk	Movement Snack	Recovery	Martial Arts	Just Move
Dance	Run	Movement Snack	Recovery	Group Exercise	Just Move
Dance	Run	Movement Snack	Recovery	Group Exercise	Just Move
Dance	Run	Movement Snack	Recovery	Group Exercise	Just Move

This page is blank because YOU are about to make something happen on the other side. Cut freely, or if you'd rather keep this book in one piece, scan the QR code or head to newmovesinmenopause.com to grab a printable PDF. Either way, you've got options. Just like in midlife.

This page is blank because YOU are about to make something happen on the other side. Cut freely, or if you'd rather keep this book in one piece, scan the QR code or head to newmovesinmenopause.com to grab a printable PDF. Either way, you've got options. Just like in midlife.

Movement Snack Icons

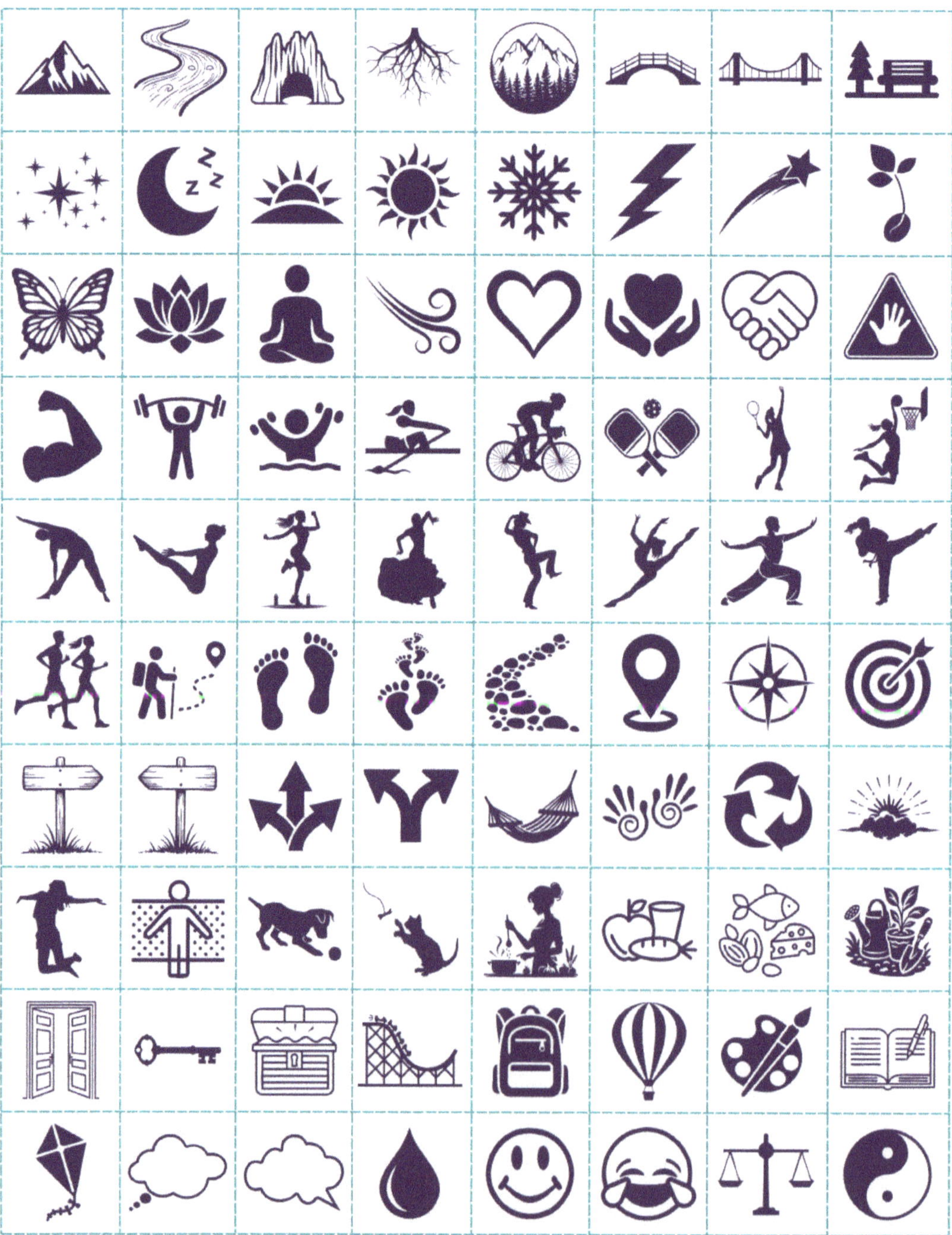

Make Your Own Icons

This page is blank because YOU are about to make something happen on the other side.
Cut freely, or if you'd rather keep this book in one piece, scan the QR code or head to
newmovesinmenopause.com to grab a printable PDF. Either way, you've got options.
Just like in midlife.

This page is blank because YOU are about to make something happen on the other side.
Cut freely, or if you'd rather keep this book in one piece, scan the QR code or head to
newmovesinmenopause.com to grab a printable PDF. Either way, you've got options.
Just like in midlife.

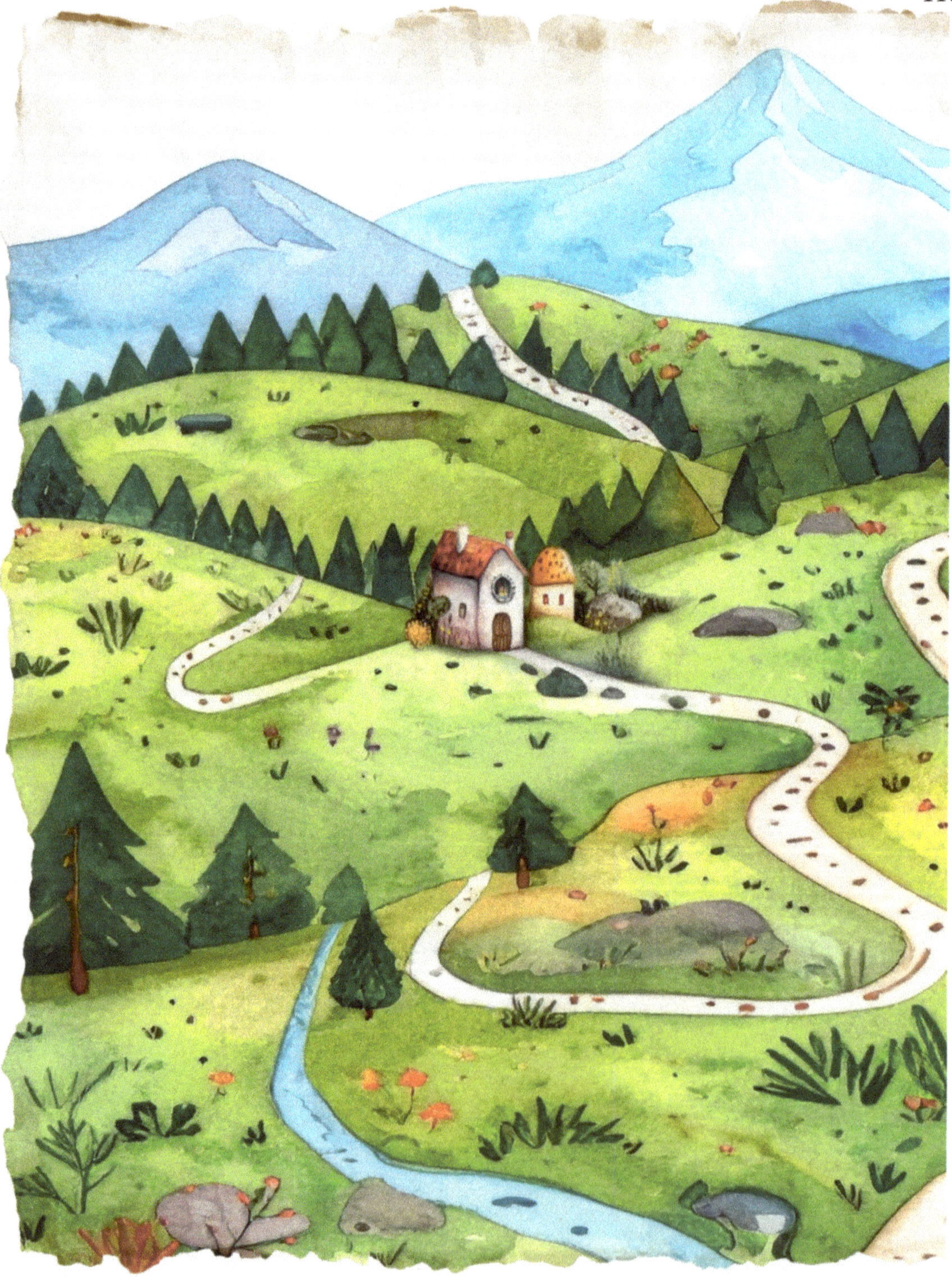

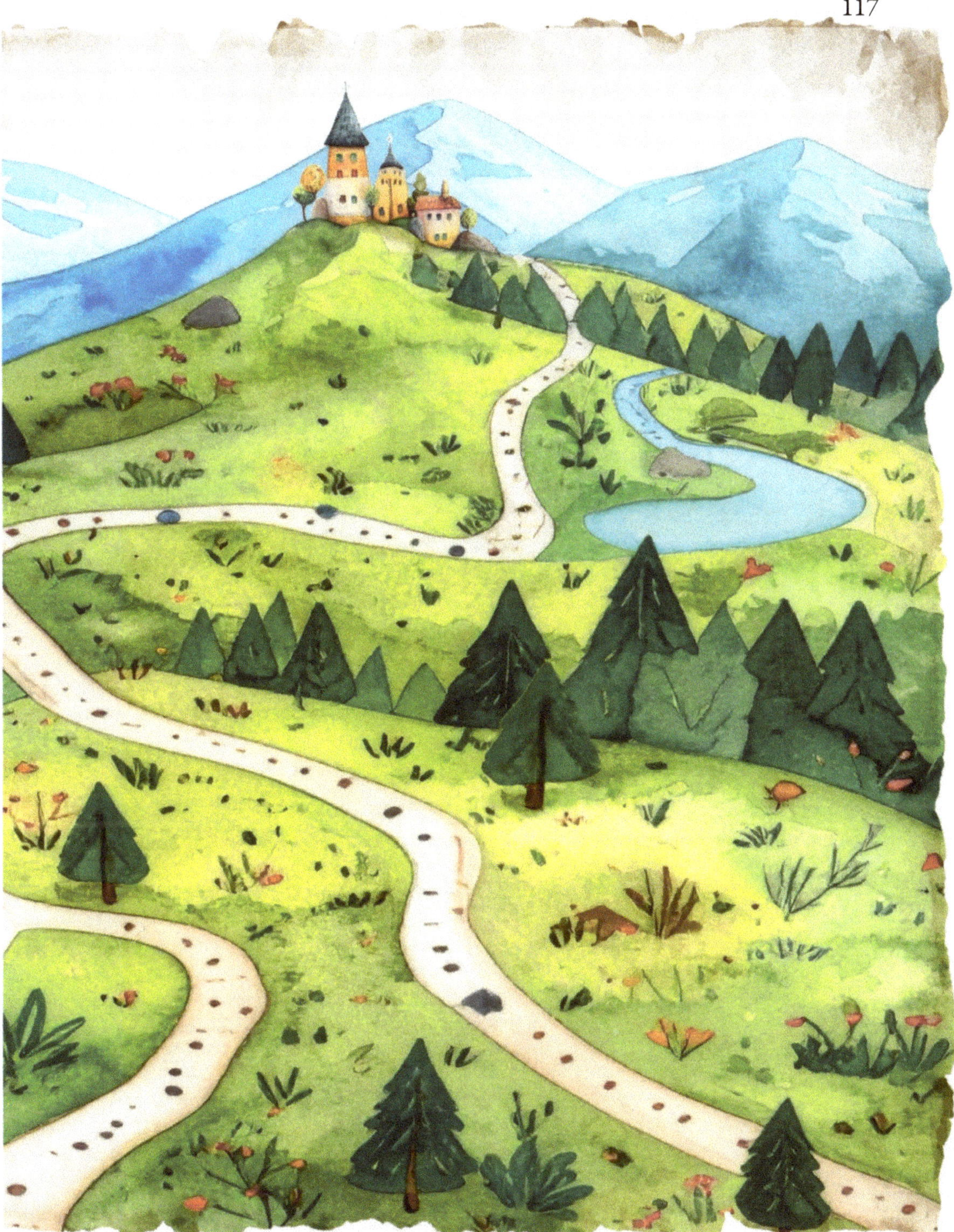

This page is blank because YOU are about to make something happen on the other side. Cut freely, or if you'd rather keep this book in one piece, scan the QR code or head to newmovesinmenopause.com to grab a printable PDF. Either way, you've got options. Just like in midlife.

This page is blank because YOU are about to make something happen on the other side.
Cut freely, or if you'd rather keep this book in one piece, scan the QR code or head to
newmovesinmenopause.com to grab a printable PDF. Either way, you've got options.
Just like in midlife.

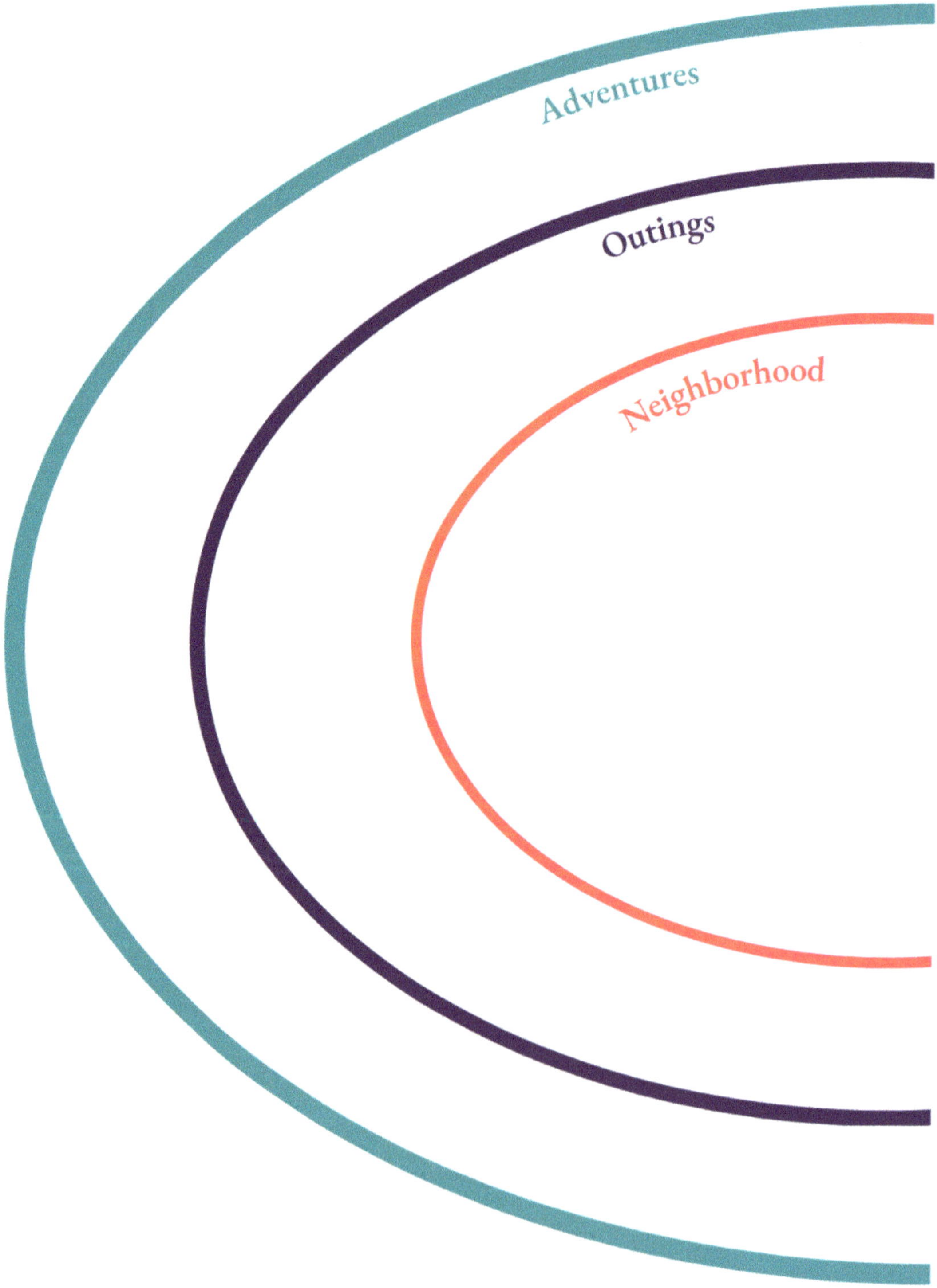

Adventures
Outings
Neighborhood

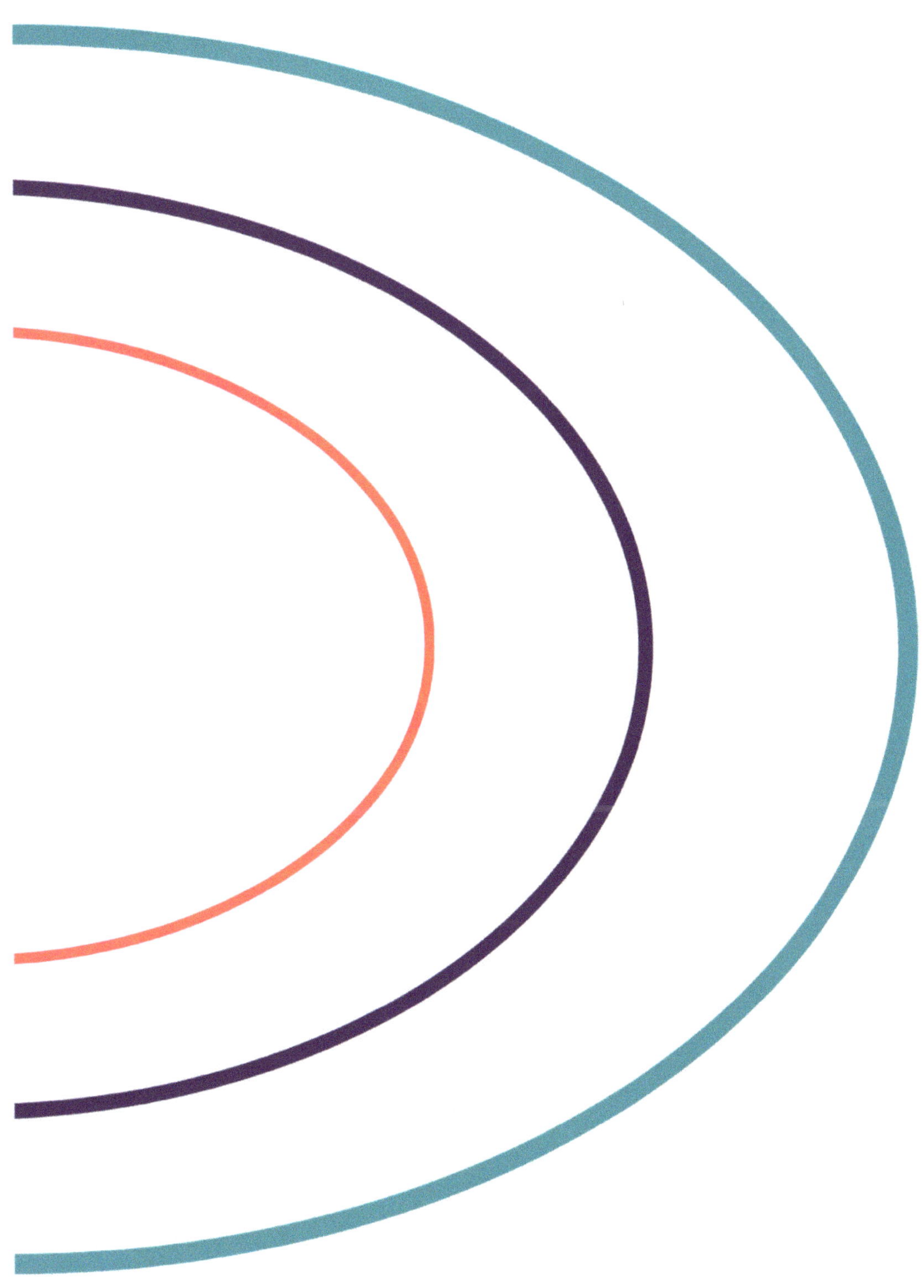

This page is blank because YOU are about to make something happen on the other side. Cut freely, or if you'd rather keep this book in one piece, scan the QR code or head to newmovesinmenopause.com to grab a printable PDF. Either way, you've got options. Just like in midlife.

This page is blank because YOU are about to make something happen on the other side. Cut freely, or if you'd rather keep this book in one piece, scan the QR code or head to newmovesinmenopause.com to grab a printable PDF. Either way, you've got options. Just like in midlife.

Adventures

Neighborho

ood

Outings

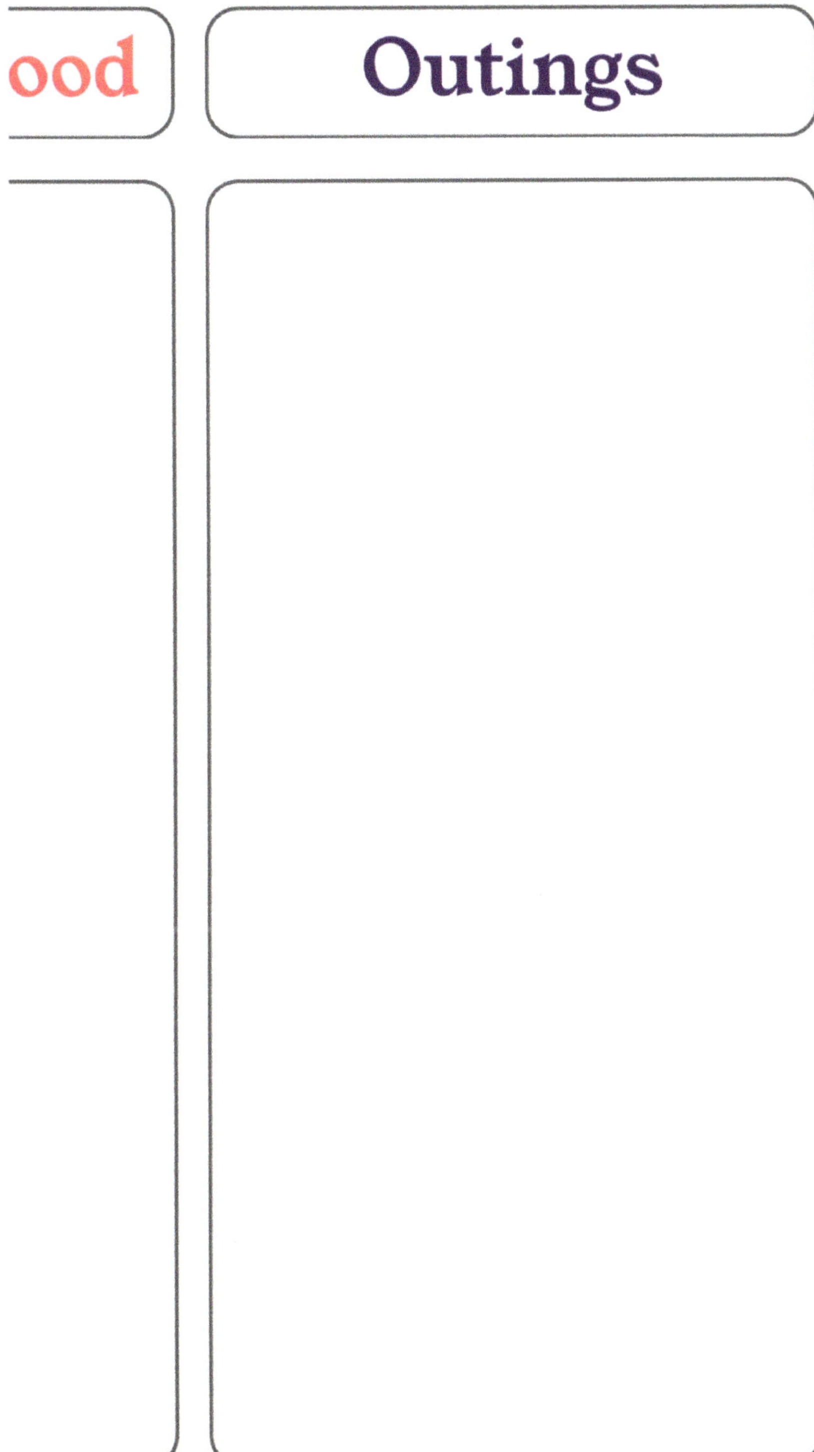

This page is blank because YOU are about to make something happen on the other side. Cut freely, or if you'd rather keep this book in one piece, scan the QR code or head to newmovesinmenopause.com to grab a printable PDF. Either way, you've got options. Just like in midlife.

Chapter 7: Motivation

It's worth repeating: When it comes to fitness, if you don't enjoy it, you won't stick with it. So let's dig a little deeper into this enjoyment factor. It sounds easy—to stay in excellent shape, just find an incredibly fun activity, and do it. A lot! But few of us get to this age without realizing that it's not that simple.

- You join a kickball league. It fits your informal, social personality. You're running around, breathing hard, drinking a beer after games, maybe even signing up for a tournament. But . . . you injure your ACL on a ski trip.
- You work your way through a couch-to-10k, self-coached training plan. You run the 10k! Next, a half-marathon. But . . . your marriage/teenage child/job suddenly becomes stressful and time-consuming. Now you no longer feel like waking up at 6 am to run. In fact, when you're asleep, you want to stay asleep.
- You've been going to the same circuit-training class forever. Suddenly, your trainer announces she's moving to Alaska. Now what? (Even though, if you're honest, you were getting just a little bored.)
- In high school, you were a competitive swimmer, so you decide to return to the pool. You've been swimming for a month now, which is good, because regular movement is good for you. The trouble is, "because it's good for me" no longer motivates you.
- You know you feel better when you're active, but for the past few months, you've been spinning your wheels. You keep signing up for classes, but nothing seems to stick. What's become of your motivation?

What, indeed. Motivation is what keeps us going after the first surge of enthusiasm begins to fade or when things don't go exactly according to plan. Understanding what motivates you—and I mean *you,* not your sister or your best friend or people you work with—is essential to customizing your movement map. I realize that social media bombards us constantly with aspirational role models, but those people are not you. (Have they even met you?) So how do you work <u>with</u>, rather than against, yourself?

A Few Things to Keep in Mind

- Motivation changes and evolves. What kept you going in your early twenties might not work for you now. Or it might need a few tweaks.

- Motivation may not be constant across all your fitness activities and goals. For example, when it comes to circuit training classes, you might discover you're a true people person who looks forward to socializing as much as working out. But you might feel completely different, about, say, a pilates class. For whatever reason, you might want to hit the reformer alone in your garage or in a setting where no one's voice is heard except the instructor's.

- It usually takes more than one kind of motivation to get us where we want to go. There's nothing wrong with that. For example, are you engaging in a particular activity because you enjoy the activity itself or are because of the way you feel during or afterwards? It could be, and more than likely is, a little of both.

- Try not to confuse motivation with obligation or guilt. What you think you *should* do is different from *how* you get yourself to do that thing. (Also, remember **should vs. good?**)

- Motivation comes in different strengths. Short-term motivation is whatever it takes to get you out the door. Long-term motivation takes some self-examination. You'll need some of each.

Types of fitness motivation

- **Better physical health** is at the top of everyone's list, which is understandable, but can also be overwhelming. How do you measure good health? Whose advice (or warnings) will you listen to?

- **Improved mental health** and stress relief—who doesn't want these?

- Most women I train say they're motivated, to varying degrees, by a desire to **improve or maintain their appearance**. Some want to look good "for their age," or skip aging altogether or recapture their "best body. " I don't have to tell you that our culture reinforces this desire. But in my experience as a trainer, this kind of motivation is hard to maintain over the long haul, especially as we get older.

- So many women express frustration when their latest fitness commitment fails to produce the results they want—usually weight loss or a "better" body. But their tone changes when they talk about how exercise makes them *feel*. The truth is that movement can dramatically improve the way you feel *in the body you have right now*. **Improved body image** is a powerful motivator.

- **Fun**. I'm going to assume you know what I mean by this!

- Menopause itself has the power to motivate, for a number of reasons:

  - At this stage, you may find that you have more time to take care of yourself, as opposed to others.

  - You may be more willing to try new things, even to take risks, from looking silly in public to speaking up when you're usually silent to trying a challenging new sport. It feels good to take a chance—once you try it, you'll probably want more of it. Life gets interesting when you care less about what other people think.

Motivation enhancers

Read through the list below and start thinking about what you prefer.

- **Morning vs. Night**. Are you a morning person? Or do you have more energy—or need more of a break—at the end of the work day? You're the best judge of your own energy cycles. Why not work out when your body and mind can make the most of it?

- **Indoors vs. outdoors**. Summer days in Texas routinely exceed 100 degrees. That's just one of the reasons I prefer to work out indoors, whether in a big box gym or my home studio. I enjoy outdoor dog walks with my daughter, but when it's time for serious weight training, I want a dedicated space where equipment is safe from the elements and I don't have to deal with mosquitoes or heat stroke. Then again, the Fitness Fairies, my longest-running boot camp group, has met outdoors for more than a decade, and that's how they like it. Again, no right or wrong, just what appeals to you.

- **Group vs. solitary workouts**. Which are energizing? Which leave you feeling drained? Remember, you can feel both ways, depending on the activity. Some of the group workout classes I teach seem fueled by gossip, but some of those same friendly, noisy women serve as their own best companions on bike rides or runs.

- **Coaching vs. self-taught.** Do you appreciate instruction, structure, having someone keep track of your progress and encourage you to keep going? Or are you happier working through training plans on your own, whether or not a coach designed them?

- **Tracking progress vs. Going with the flow**. Do you feel inspired by logging your workouts? Or do you prefer to treat them as a time to *be here now.* Or is it a combination of the two?

- **Competition vs. No Way!** Does competition make movement more interesting—whether you're pitting yourself against other athletes in a formal setting or yourself in your back yard or home gym? Or does it have the power to make you lose interest altogether?

Exploration: Movement Enhancers (Example)

Morning ——————————————————✗——— Night

How it's working for me: *Early morning boot-camp classes are practical, but I never feel awake enough to go. No wonder I spend more time skating at the roller rink, at night, when that disco ball really twinkles.*

Inside ————✗————————————————— Outside

How it's working for me: *It sounds crazy, but on a normal weekday, I'd rather ride the bike at the gym while watching a video of the outdoors than go to the trouble of actually riding out there, with the traffic and weather.*

Group —————————————✗——————— Solitary

How it's working for me: *Hmmm, I'm an interesting case. I would ever-so-slightly prefer not to be alone during movement, but I'm talking about one or at most two other people—good friends, ideally. Semi-private workouts with a trainer would be good (and more affordable, too).*

Coaching ——✗————————————————— Self-Taught

How it's working for me: *I don't want to become an expert in, say, foam rolling. So I watch a different Youtube video every time. Easy peasy.*

Tracking Progress ———✗———————————— Go with the Flow

How it's working for me: *I love the pedometer on my phone. I love the way the miles add up, especially when I'm walking to explore rather than to get a workout in.*

Competition —————————————————✗— No Way!

How it's working for me: *My friend invited me to join her on that app that lets you log mileage and compete with other local people at your sport of choice. She said I'd love it. I don't, because . . . well, does it matter? The point is, I deleted the app and looked for something based more on entertainment than competition. That's how I found the Zombies, Run! App. It lets me pretend I'm running through a post-apocalyptic emergency, coming to the rescue of civilization. (Check it out!)*

Exploration: Movement Enhancers

Read over the list of motivation binaries below (and the next page). Grab a colored pencil and mark an X on the line in the approximate place you belong. Below that, write about a time when embracing your motivation preference helped you in a physical fitness activity.

Morning ———————————————————————— Night
How it's working for me:

Inside ———————————————————————— Outside
How it's working for me:

Group ———————————————————————— Solitary
How it's working for me:

Coaching ——————————————————————— Self-Taught
How it's working for me:

Tracking Progress ————————————————— Go with the Flow
How it's working for me:

Competition ——————————————————————— No Way!
How it's working for me:

Motivation killers

- Every workout can't be wildly entertaining, but if you're truly **bored**, there's no point in trying harder to show up for something that's stopped working for you. Maybe it's time for a change.

- **Body Shaming**. "You should be in better shape at this point in your life." "If you don't work out every day, you're ignoring your own health." "You shouldn't leave the house till you throw out those ratty workout clothes and get more flattering ones." No matter who's delivering these messages—a doctor, an "expert", your own inner critic—they're not good for you. They're both ineffective and meanspirited. The only thing they'll motivate you to do is give up.

- **Making the perfect the enemy of the good.** Unrealistic, rigid standards are the typical culprits here. Expecting to constantly surpass yourself—to never make a mistake—is a recipe for discouragement. Instead, find small (even tiny) victories to celebrate. If you ask me, just showing up qualifies as a win.

- **Letting the past veto the present.** Just because your body looked, or performed, a certain way twenty years ago is no reason to try—over and over again, mostly without success—to recapture that moment in time. Is there another part of your life you would expect never to change?

- **Buying into empty promises.** Okay, so maybe you're tempted by the branded "cleanse" promoted by a movie star. (I put quote marks around "cleanse" because your intestinal tract does a good job of cleaning itself.) I think most of us realize that none of these miracle cures work, but some of us are seduced anyway. Why? Because suspending disbelief, even for a few days, allows you to surrender responsibility for your own health and well-being. But sooner or later, you have to admit it was all a dream. This cycle is terrible for motivation.

- **Putting your own needs last**. A lot of us are caretakers of one kind or another, always having our fitness plans derailed by sudden schedule changes, real emergencies, or any number of other obligations. The key, I think, is to expect the disruption. Remind yourself that your mental and physical health is as important as anyone else's.

- **Illness or injury.** They don't discriminate! Sooner or later, we all have to recuperate from something. Having to take time off doesn't make you a failure, and the healing process doesn't really pose a threat to your lifelong fitness. So don't get discouraged; get comfortable. Take care of yourself. Ask for help and start back small.

Exploration: Motivation Killers

Read over the motivation killers below. Grab a colored pencil and circle anything you've experienced during your movement journey. (Circle all three or just one or two—you do you!) In the table below anything you've circled, briefly describe how this killer showed up, and come up with ideas for neutralizing the killer in the future. Here's an example:

BODY SHAMING

Enter the killer:	Neutralizing strategies:
I told myself I was disgusting because I couldn't fit into my favorite jeans. Decided to buy a Fitbit and let it show me how to lose weight and get fit. Never used the Fitbit, so I couldn't tell you if it works.	*Apologize to myself for that nasty language! Collect evidence that I'm the opposite of disgusting—adorable, majestic, delectable? Sell the Fitbit on Craigslist, use the proceeds to buy jeans that fit. Wear those jeans to the nearest pickleball court and learn to play.*

Your turn...

BODY SHAMING

Enter the killer:	Neutralizing strategies:

BOREDOM

Enter the killer:	Neutralizing strategies:

LETTING PERFECT BE THE ENEMY OF GOOD

Enter the killer:	Neutralizing strategies:

Exploration: I Want to . . . But . . .

Spend a few moments reviewing what you learned about yourself from the Motivation Enhancers and Motivation Killers explorations. Remind yourself of what gets you going–and what stops, slows you down to a crawl.

If you like, write a short summary of your motivation style.
Example: *I like to go on scavenger hunts, expeditions, pathfinding—anything where I get to follow a mysterious path and have an adventure. I do NOT like to be given a detailed plan—I react as if it's a list of horrible household chores. I rebel.*

Now, think of three types of movement that either
- Interest you, but you haven't managed to do
- You once did and enjoyed, but for whatever reason, stopped
- These activities can be big or small—anything from "run a marathon" to "walk to happy hour."

1.

2.

3.

Now, using the list of motivation enhancers, use your natural motivation style to get closer to these goals. You can do this on the next page.

Here's an example:
I want to: *try aqua aerobics*
But: *I haven't even found a pool*
Motivation-based fix: *The idea of signing on to a rigid schedule and chatting with strangers in a pool is freaking me out a little. But the thing is, my neighbor has a pool. I wonder if there's any such thing as a video water aerobics class? Turns out there is!*

I want to:

But:

Motivation-based fixes:

I want to:

But:

Motivation-based fixes:

I want to:

But:

Motivation-based fixes:

A few strategies that seem to work for everyone

Carpool accountability is simple. If you want to increase the odds that you'll show up for a planned movement activity, ask if anyone needs a ride. Or ask if someone will pick you up. You've just doubled your odds of attendance!

Variation 1: Ask if anyone wants to walk or bike or take mass transit, agree on a time, and show up!

Variation 2: Agree to meet someone—for a swim, a walk, a class—at a certain time and place. For some reason, most of us are far more dependable when another person gets involved. To put it another way, even if we have a habit of bailing on ourselves, we're much less likely to bail on our friends.

Variation 3 (for introverts): Make a plan to do some kind of scheduled movement practice—alone! Take before and after selfies as proof you followed through and to remind you of how much fun you did (or didn't) have.

This is the perfect time to add some carpool accountability to your movement map. You might do this by designing your own icon, or by writing a big **C.A.** next to an activity that qualifies, or . . . .

Movement as a 24-hour buffet

A lot of people I meet assume I stick to a perfectly disciplined routine at the gym. They might be surprised to learn what an improviser I've become. Sometimes I'll spend several weeks doing nothing but full-body workouts. I'll then switch to a split routine where I train my upper- or lower-body on alternate days. Some days I go to the gym with a plan in mind, only to throw it out in favor of some high-impact, high-intensity bouncy stuff. As for cardio, some weeks it's nothing but short walks squeezed in between meetings. But then, especially if I'm listening to a new audiobook, I'll shift into a season of much longer walks—45 minutes at a minimum.

I've given myself a lot of options and so should you. Why commit to an expensive 5-course meal when you could pick and choose, depending on your appetite and mood?

I have clients who go through phases and enthusiasms in a yearly cycle—swimming in summer, playing league soccer in the fall. It's okay to switch activities. It might even be better for your body—the more variety, the less likelihood of a repetitive injury.

That's the big picture approach to the **buffet of movement.** You can also tune into your appetites on a daily or even hourly basis. If you wake up uninspired by the prospect of going to your habitual class at the gym, that's okay. You have options. What else is going on at the gym today? Wanna try that instead? How's the weather? Could you do something outdoors? The point is, you get to decide. Give yourself free rein.

And on days when you feel lazy, uninspired, or pulled in a million directions, enjoy a few **Movement Snacks**—little bites of activity that add up over time. In my life, that might look like a few squats during a Zoom meeting, stretching between clients, or a quick dance break with my daughter while dinner's cooking.

"Legalizing" snacks and repeated trips through the buffet line opens up new possibilities, as this letter from a client shows:

Hey Maria, sometimes I'm uninspired by the sight of my home gym. All the gear is nice, but where are my buddies? Who will bring the gossip? What if I just don't want to be indoors? Luckily, I have options. Today, I'm just gonna snack:

- *15 minutes of resistance training in my home gym, even though that sounds boring, because I'll listen to AC/DC as loud as possible!*

- *15 more minutes of cleaning my home gym. It'll involve a lot of picking weights up and putting them down, as well as some flexibility and mobility (and shop-vaccing).*

- *20 minutes digging up a new garden bed, moving several large rocks in the process. It's hot out, so 20 very sweaty minutes.*

- *15 minutes of running around in the park with my grandson. I didn't say "sprinting" but I didn't say "strolling," either.*

You'll find a selection of Movement Snack icons on pages 112-113. I recommend sprinkling them all over your map!

Let's talk about goals

We live in a world obsessed with goals: 10,000 steps, 30-day challenges, five-year plans. Goals can give us direction, structure, and for some of us, a little dopamine hit when we hit a benchmark. Goals can turn vague desires (*"I want to feel better"*) into actions. And that's powerful . . . when used wisely.

But all goals aren't created equal, and not all seasons require them.

Goals work beautifully when they're rooted in your current beliefs, values, and preferences. In midlife, from what I've seen, goals based on *how you want to feel* rather than *how you think you should look* are the most effective. Sometimes that's a matter of word choice:

At our first meeting, Christine announced her goal—to "get back to her old self," which meant a marathon-running, 5 a.m.-gym-going version of herself from 10 years ago. But between work, caregiving, and a body that was clearly in a new phase, that goal was producing more frustration than fuel. So we talked, quite a bit, about how she pictured her "old self" interacting with her present life. It turned out she didn't really want to run another marathon—in fact, she decided she'd rather spend time with her kids than find someone to watch them while she ran. Her new goal became "to build stamina for long hikes with my children." Same desire for endurance, but the meaning changed and with it, her motivation.

Goals backfire when they start *running* your life without improving your *quality* of life.

Lauren came to her first session armed with color-coded spreadsheets, each for a different goal. There was a column for diet, exercise (with subcategories for cardio, resistance training, HIIT, and yoga), and sleep. She wanted me to help her set a target for each. At first, I was elated—I love a client who's already done her homework! Before long, though, I realized her life was being constantly monitored by three different fitness apps, tracking everything from macros to workouts to sleep. Yes, they reminded her (24/7) to take the next step. No, this didn't leave time for Lauren to have anything approaching a satisfying life. I began to think that whatever benefit she'd gotten from her goals started to wear off. She'd lost touch with her own internal cues. She wasn't listening to her body.

So one day, during a session, I asked how her body felt in that moment. She froze! I could see that she didn't understand what I meant. At that point, our work became about reconnecting her mind to her body, like repairing a circuit that disconnected from years of "doing,"pushing," and "counting."

I instituted "goal-less" movement days, when the only aim was to notice what felt good. I suggested she keep a journal to write down how she felt after movement—not how long or how many reps she did, but how she felt. Thirty days in, Lauren identified a pattern: she loved being outdoors with friends, whether hiking, playing pickleball, or going for a bike ride around town that ended with a burger and fries. Every other weekend, she reserved time for "goal-less joy" on her calendar and made plans to spend active time with friends, preferably outdoors. She was surprised to discover that she felt less stressed out about all the fitness boxes still to be checked. She still checked them off when she remembered, but she'd stopped pressuring herself.

When we become so focused on *achieving* that we forget to *experience*, the goal has lost its purpose. Setting goals around mindfulness, for instance, just doesn't work. If you're constantly measuring how "in the moment" you are, the moment has left the building. I've also observed a tipping point at which sticking with a goal becomes less about growth and more about ego—the running schedule that punishes your knees or the diet that's sucked all the spice out of your life but "worked in the past."

Letting go of a goal doesn't always equal quitting. It's recalibrating. Finding a better, easier path.

And here's a radical thought: some goals deserve to be abandoned. Maybe it's time for a goal audit. Midlife is the perfect time.

Ask yourself:

- Is this goal serving me, or am I serving it?

- Does it align with what matters to me *today*?

- Does it make me feel free or trapped?

Sometimes, the most meaningful progress isn't measured in metrics but in moments: waking up with more energy, laughing more freely, or feeling at peace in your own skin. A good goal points you toward something meaningful, but it should also leave room for detours, rest stops, and dance breaks along the way.

Chapter 8: Nourishment

First, A BIG DISCLAIMER.

My perspective on bodyweight, nutrition and food is weight-and-size neutral, for reasons I hope will become crystal clear. That said, discussions of weight, health, diet, culture, and even nutrition can be triggering for some people. If you're one of those people, you may want to skip this.

Also, I'm neither a registered dietitian nor a nutritionist, but a fitness trainer. I'm not an expert, but the resources chapter can direct you to several. That said, most of my clients are hungry for information about how to nourish their bodies and how to untangle conflicting messages about their bodies' weight and size. I've noticed that menopause adds a layer of anxiety. So I try to keep up with the research and find out what answers I can. Along the way, I've developed . . . well, I guess you could call it a philosophy.

Speaking of which, please take a moment to notice what this chapter *isn't* called:

- Nutrition in Menopause, with specific metrics and targets for women in midlife.

- You eat too much of the wrong kind of food.

- You don't eat enough of the right kind of food.

Again, this chapter is NOT ABOUT ANY OF THE ABOVE, even though women in menopause supposedly have a bottomless appetite for these topics. (That's what social media tells me.) Most of us are only a click or two away from food advice that promises unbelievable results.

- Limit calories to ___ per day: lose two pounds per week.

- Eliminate entire food groups: cure health problems, lose weight, live forever.

- Balance your hormones by eating (or not eating) very specific foods.

- Here's the secret "cleanse" that will rid your body of "toxins." (Your body doesn't need a detox plan, it *is* a detox plan, courtesy of your organs. Unless you've been snacking on poisonous stuff, your liver's already got your back.)

Of course, practically no one can actually follow this kind of "advice" for long, and, not surprisingly, there's no research to back it up. Whoever is selling this stuff seems to believe that:

- Women are pretty much the same—they need the same amount and the same types of food and nutrients.

- We need to "get control" of our food.

- Food (and our appetite for it) is the enemy.

While I believe that what you eat can improve your quality of life in menopause to some extent, I distrust messaging that extols certain foods as miracles and others as poison. I wish more fitness authorities talked about food in a real way.

You know what? I'll start.

My life with food

I grew up in a Spanish village, where everyone's life revolved around food, in the form of three meals each day, all eaten sitting down with the family. We ate what I now think of as *peasant food*—home-grown vegetables and meat, simple preparations, big celebrations revolving around feasts, and local red wine. (And maybe a glass of *'digestivo'* after dinner!) Essentially, it's the Mediterranean diet, Spanish version. To this day, everything people eat in my home village is fresh and unprocessed. Everyone has a garden; everyone sits down to eat together. On Sunday afternoons, people come by my parents' house to eat—nothing fancy, just whatever guests bring and whatever's in my mother's kitchen. My aunt usually brings a *roscon*, a sort of bundt cake, my mom busts out the bread, ham, chorizo and salchichon, all made on our uncle's farm, and big pots of tea and coffee. These meals go on all afternoon. The volume and depth of the gossip always amazes me—after all, these are people who see and speak to each other every day! When my parents visit me in the US, my mother always packs her paella pan.

I know it sounds pleasantly relaxed, but my sister and I were definitely expected to obey certain food rules. You finished every morsel on your plate or you didn't leave the table! (My mother had grown up with 17 brothers and sisters, and money was extremely tight, so when she said, "You don't know what hunger is," I believed her.)

So, did I internalize this healthy relationship with food and sail into adulthood without the slightest body-image trouble? Well, not exactly. I've always been athletic, equating all kinds of movement with fun. As for food, I liked it, I ate it, I didn't stress about it. But growing up, leaving home and moving to the US changed my relationship with food.

My low point came in the late 1990s. Stuck in a bad marriage and desperate to lose myself in something, I got serious about strength-training—or, more accurately, bodybuilding. This quickly became a means of control, over the size and shape of my muscles, but also over my emotions, and certainly over food. Determined to get bigger, I ate strictly for physical results, barely tasting the food. It was typical bodybuilder behavior—the more control you exert, the better your results. I certainly got positive feedback about my appearance. Which meant I was doing well, succeeding, seeing results. I was also miserably unhappy. In case you wonder, looking at my "best body ever" in the mirror didn't improve my mood.

Here's what I learned: Controlling your body's size and composition through food and exercise is not the key to a satisfying life. Yes, you'll be told the opposite. Don't believe it.

Fast forward twenty-plus years. I'm still very athletic. I still enjoy a wide variety of physical activity, with strength training at its core. I no longer move to achieve a goal—to get bigger, for instance, or to lose weight. I try to make the most of my food, from a nutritional standpoint, but never at the cost of enjoyment. (Can you believe I used to eat boiled chicken with brown rice and broccoli every single day?) These days, my food has to taste good—no, great! I love experimenting with new recipes. Raising a daughter has intensified my commitment not just to healthy eating, but to a healthy relationship with food.

I occasionally keep track of certain metrics, such as whether or not I'm getting adequate protein. I go through food phases that might strike you as eccentric—tuna/hotdog curry with ketchup, anyone? But I'm okay with myself, and that's what matters. At the moment, I'm not as lean as I once was. Like many women in their fifties, I've accumulated a bit of abdominal fat. I remind myself, as many times as possible, that this isn't a sign of failure, but simply where my body needs to be right now. Meanwhile, I'm enjoying the joy and connection food brings to my life. I'm healthier and happier than I've ever been, and this little belly of mine doesn't change that one bit!

Body image issues come up for me fairly regularly, as they do for just about all my clients, but I don't blame food, because food is no longer my enemy, but my BFF. I pride myself on being able to turn anything into a taco—leftover fish from last night's dinner, rotisserie chicken, rice and beans . . . I could eat you every day!

Numbers, measurements, metrics

When I started out as a trainer, many years ago, I kept data on my clients—everything from body weight to measurements, body-fat percentages and improvements in reps and weight lifted. Clients seemed to expect this kind of record-keeping. They found it motivational, in the short run. The long run, though, was another story. No one can keep making astounding progress forever. What if you get sick, go on vacation, have a baby?

I began to think that long-lasting fitness improvements don't come from metrics, but almost in spite of them. After all, so many number-based goals are attached to appearance, and while there's nothing wrong with liking the way you look, health and wellbeing are so much more important. I also believe that healthy doesn't look a certain way.

Some of my clients already know this. Some need a little gentle persuasion to step away from the scale and the calipers and start thinking about how food impacts their quality of life.

***

Okay. Let's talk about the elephant in the room. Everyone wants to **lose weight,** it seems. If my clients don't mention weight loss as their primary goal, it's certainly a desirable outcome. Even if they're tired of yoyo dieting, they believe they *should* lose weight. They've heard that Americans are the stars of the obesity epidemic. They want, in a general way, to be healthier—and weight loss and improved health are said to go hand in hand. Google *sprained ankles, high blood pressure, migraine headaches* or *osteoporosis* and you'll be advised to "achieve or maintain a healthy weight," as if all healing begins with weight loss.

Well, I'm sorry, but weight loss is not simple. Here's what research tells us:

- Fewer than 1% of the millions of people who diet are able to lose weight and keep it off. Multiple studies have shown that "more than half of the lost weight was regained within two years, and by five years, more than 80% of lost weight was regained."

- What exactly is a "healthy weight?" Height-weight tables and the BMI are outdated. They don't take into account cardiovascular fitness, metabolic health (how efficient your body turns what you eat into the energy your body needs), muscle mass, bone density, age, sex, ethnicity, or fat distribution.

- Weight is not an accurate indicator of health. Studies demonstrate that focusing on weight alone ignores such determinants of health as physical activity, nutrition, blood markers, and mental well-being.

- Dieting is a predictable gateway to eating disorders.

- People who diet repeatedly are at a much higher risk for obesity than people who don't diet at all. Even one intentional weight loss episode is associated with a doubled risk of becoming overweight.

Everything on that list is substantiated by rigorous research. But despite the compelling evidence that diets don't work, weight loss is still seen as the gold standard for getting healthy and fit.

You can thank **diet culture** for keeping this message in regular rotation. It's been going strong for decades; it's alive and well today. Most Americans—especially female Americans—are constantly being invited to give dieting another try. And another try. And yet another. So many of my clients struggle to undo the mindset of trying another diet, something that "worked for them in the past," never mind that, like most diets, it didn't work for long. The diets vary—from low-fat to keto to intermittent fasting to biohacking and carb-cycling—but the message doesn't. And neither does the research, but who cares, because there's definitely a profit to be made!

As if that weren't bad enough, there's also a big shaming campaign at play here. As long as we're *trying to diet, working on it,* signing back up, we're worthy of respect, whereas anyone who consciously opts out of this silliness is not. You may not think you've been subject to this kind of pressure, but it's insidious. Much of diet culture is internalized. Maybe it's time to listen to what you say to yourself, even subconsciously. Do you describe yourself as *fat, disgusting, out-of-control, huge, being either "good" or "bad?"*

Don't do that. It doesn't help. It hurts. Step away.

If you're serious about living a long, fit, healthy life in menopause, start questioning whether or not you "should" lose a few pounds. Should you, really?nd will my barking that order at you make it so?

How much of your mental energy has been taken up with weight loss so far? How much more are you willing to give?

What about weight loss drugs?

GLP-1 agonist medications are a significant—and very new—development. You almost certainly know someone who's taking Ozempic, Wegovy, Mounjaro, or one of the others, and you've certainly seen the ads. You may be considering trying a GLP-1 yourself.

My clients ask me about GLP-1 medications all the time, and here's how I respond—this isn't my area of expertise, and I'm not here to tell anyone what to do with their body. Hopefully, you have a trusted medical professional to guide you through that. I'm not your mother! I'm not here to judge.

And I'll be honest—GLP-1s have been a genuine game-changer. The medical establishment has finally had to admit that the "comprehensive lifestyle intervention" approach they've been promoting for decades hasn't worked very well. These new drugs have produced remarkable results for those with type 2 diabetes and other conditions linked to excess weight.

The weight loss some people experience can also act as a powerful catalyst. When exercise is no longer seen as punishment for eating or a weight loss tool, movement can finally be about strength and joy. That's a huge shift—and a good one.

But I also have concerns. These drugs were designed for very specific populations: individuals with type 2 diabetes or obesity who didn't respond to lifestyle interventions. The effortless weight loss that followed made headlines, and soon the story became less about health and more about aesthetics. Now, people are taking these drugs for cosmetic reasons, often without medical necessity. These days an army of unqualified influencers is pushing GLP-1s to anyone with a pulse and a scale, promising to melt off those "last stubborn five pounds" or stop weight gain before it starts. It's giving big *"start Botox before you get wrinkles"* energy. Fear marketing at its finest.

It's important to remember that weight loss doesn't equal fat loss. Despite decades of promises from the diet and fitness industries, spot reduction simply doesn't exist. No cream, crunch, or injection can tell your body *where* to lose fat—it's just not how biology works. If you lose muscle—and most people do during rapid weight loss—you're not just lighter, you're weaker. When the weight inevitably returns after stopping the medication, it often comes back as fat, not muscle. For women in menopause, that's a real concern. We're already facing the double whammy of declining bone density and age-related muscle loss—and since muscle protects bone, losing it only makes things worse.

If you're considering GLP-1 medications, please **prioritize resistance training.** And **get a DEXA scan** before you start and **regularly** thereafter, so you can monitor any muscle loss. (These scans also track bone density—good information to have.)

Thoughts on healthy eating

You know how when you meet someone and instantly think, "Ah, she gets it"? That's how I feel about Dr. Jenn Salib-Huber. She is an internationally known registered dietitian and naturopathic doctor who helps women in midlife cut through the confusion and feel at home in their changing bodies. We first connected on Instagram and later as a guest on her podcast. Her approach to food is everything I love—intuitive, realistic, and grounded in self-care, not restriction. I'm thrilled she agreed to share her thoughts on healthy eating. This is what she had to say:

> Rather than focusing on counting calories, I recommend strategies that align with intuitive eating and the Health at Every Size (HAES) framework. These approaches help women avoid the pitfalls of diet culture and disordered eating, while supporting the behaviours associated with better health in midlife and menopause. As I like to remind the women I work with, we can only control the behaviours we choose, not the outcome of those behaviours.

> 1. **Add more plants to your plate**
>   A plant-forward approach to menopause nutrition, especially one that includes plant-based protein from beans and lentils, offers a powerhouse combo of fiber, protein, and phytoestrogens that can help ease menopausal symptoms and support overall metabolic health. It's also in line with the Mediterranean pattern of eating, which is recommended for women in menopause.

> 2. **Feed your muscles well, but don't obsess over protein**
>   Prioritizing satisfying protein at meals and snacks helps maintain lean muscle and supports steady energy and satiety. Plan to include "main character" protein sources throughout the day,

such as beans, Greek yogurt, tofu, meat, eggs and fish. But try to remember that protein isn't magical, and can't work by itself.

3. **Love your gut.**
   Fiber-rich foods such as berries, beans, lentils, and whole grains help keep you full and satisfied, support healthy digestion, blood-sugar balance, and heart health. They won't "blast belly fat," but they do help your body thrive.

4. **Add before you subtract.**
   Instead of obsessing over what to remove, think about simple add-ins that make meals more colorful, nourishing, and satisfying, like extra veggies in your pasta sauce, or a sprinkle of nuts and seeds on your morning yogurt. For most women, nutrition by addition will always win over restriction.

5. **Build strength you can see and feel.**
   Move toward pleasurable, sustainable physical activity. Resistance training is one of the most powerful ways to protect muscle and metabolism as we age, and research shows it can also reduce visceral fat even without weight loss. Instead of letting the scale dictate your success in the gym, notice how your confidence builds alongside your strength.

I love Dr. Jenn's advice. I'll add just a few things I've learned from my clients.

- **Learn about intuitive eating,** mindful eating or any other philosophy that encourages you to slow down and experience food in the moment. You'll become more aware of your hunger and fullness signals, what foods you truly enjoy, and how different foods make your body feel. My friend Katherine points out that it's not something you learn, but something you remember. "You know how kids take an eternity to eat a single spaghetti strand? How they examine it, slap it on different body parts to see how it feels, before putting it in their mouth and only then deciding whether it's pleasant or not? While we may not eat like a child in the moment, we can become more child-like in the enjoyment of our food." A word of caution: be suspicious of any intuition-based food plan that promises weight loss. Sometimes a more conscious approach to eating has that result, but it's not really the point.

- Remember the **Blue Zone people?** Those hundred-year-old longevity experts have a few food behaviors in common. They tend to eat locally produced, minimally processed food and they usually sit at a table crowded with friends and family. Big celebrations, usually involving local wine, are held throughout the year. And they eat three times as many vegetables as people in most first-world nations. Talk about adding not subtracting!

- **If you're the kind of person who classifies food as either good or bad, stop it,** because that attitude does nothing to improve your health. Some food is more nutritious than other food, but there's no point in shaming yourself over food choices, and, as we've already discussed, diets that try to eliminate "bad foods" fail miserably.

- **Menopause changes everything,** so don't be surprised if it changes the way your body reacts to food. For instance, hormonal shifts can make some women newly sensitive to familiar foods. Keeping a food journal can be a great way to identify foods that cause problems—but food journals can also be a sneaky way to obsess over your diet or your weight, so be careful.

The top four nutrition questions I'm asked, even though I'm not a nutritionist: Protein—should I be eating more?

This one's been at the top of the charts as far back as I can remember, but as I write this, it's really having a moment.

So, here's the deal:yes, protein matters. It's essential for muscle repair, strength, metabolism, and satiety. But that doesn't justify the current Not Enough Protein Panic. I've found that, with a bit of awareness, intentionality, and a few nutritional tweaks, women can reach their daily recommended amounts without having to turn every meal into a math problem. Simply remembering to include a source of protein at each meal or snack makes a huge difference.

For most women in midlife, a good target is 1.2–1.6 grams of protein per kilogram of body weight per day. *Per kilogram,* not per pound! A 150-pound woman needs roughly 80-110 grams of protein per day.

Can fasted workouts help me lose fat?

Here's my honest take—Maybe? I don't know if this (or any other diet strategy) is going to help you lose weight. The jury is still out about intermittent fasting. But if you'd rather not eat before you workout, go for it.

From a physiological standpoint, working out fasted may slightly increase fat oxidation *during* the workout, but total fat loss over time depends more on overall nutrition and training consistency. For most women, performance and recovery matter more than squeezing out that theoretical "fat-burning" edge.

If you feel great training fasted, keep doing it. If you feel sluggish or hungry, don't fast. Eat something small (a banana, a piece of toast with nut butter) before you work out.

Most importantly, listen to your body, not TikTok trends.

How worried should I be about added sugar?

Sugar is currently one of the top villains in the nutrition multiverse. Predictably, the conversation has gotten *way* too black-and-white.

Here's the truth: your body can handle sugar. What it struggles with is chronic overconsumption, which can be blamed (somewhat) on the sugar hidden in processed foods, sweetened drinks, and snacks you don't even think of as sweet. That's the stuff to keep an eye on, because it can quietly add up and displace more nutrient-dense foods.

But let's not throw joy out with the frosting. Sharing a slice of your kid's birthday cake, celebrating with dessert on date night, or enjoying an occasional splash of whipped cream on your coffee (oh yes please)—none of that rises to the level of overconsumption.

Sugar shouldn't become a moral battleground.

Yes, Big Food is not entirely trustworthy, but no, you're not powerless against it. The key is awareness, not obsession. It helps you choose where your sugar comes from so you can enjoy it more intentionally. One cupcake never broke a metabolism, but constant guilt about it might break your spirit.

What about alcohol? Is any amount of it okay?

If you look purely at the data, there's no amount of alcohol that improves health outcomes. In other words, alcohol isn't good for you. It's a toxin your body has to process.

That said, there's more to good health than biological processes; it also involves psychology and social connection. For some of us, the occasional glass of wine or cocktail can be part of a balanced, healthy life.

News flash: I am not affiliated with The Food Police

I can't tell you how many times I've been at a party and someone, plate in hand, starts defending what she's about to eat before I've even said hello. "I know, I know, this is bad for me," "I swear, this is my cheat day," or my personal favorite: "You don't eat stuff like this, right?"

They're too busy confessing their sins to notice what's on *my* plate—usually chips smothered in queso, along with any dessert involving fruit and whipped cream. (Yes, I do eat stuff like that.) It's a blatant case of mistaken identity! I am not now, nor have I ever been, nor will I ever be, interested in joining the Food Police! I don't go to parties to judge other people's plates. Ever.

I don't mean to yell, but how else can I drown out the deep, cultural guilt we've been taught to feel about consuming food?

Chapter 9: I'll Leave You With This

Stop chasing squirrels.

For years, I was the human version of my golden retrievers, GG and Luna. Every time a shiny new trend sprinted across my field of vision—a new workout method, a "revolutionary" recovery gadget, a supplement that promised better sleep, more energy, or bigger muscles—I bolted, tail wagging, determined to hunt down perfection and catch it, once and for all.

Which, of course, never happened, anymore than GG and Luna ever caught a squirrel, no matter how fast they ran. The amazing thing is that they don't spiral about it. My dogs don't wake up the next morning questioning their worth or vowing to"do better." They're just being dogs—fully present, fully themselves, happily chasing squirrels they will never catch, and suffering zero emotional fallout.

But me? I'm human. I have a choice to make about what to chase and what not to chase. It's not always easy.

The tricky thing about squirrels is that they're everywhere and they're fast. Some of them are pretty convincing. They use scientific-sounding language. They post before-and-after photos. They swear their "3-minute morning method" is capable of changing my hormones, my moods—possibly my entire existence.

I call it The Squirrel Effect, and while it might constitute play time for a dog, it's frantic and reactive for humans like me. If I'm not careful, I'll end up darting from one distraction to the next, certain that the next darting mammal I see holds the answer.

It's hard not to look. I get it. I used to be the queen of "Ooh, maybe that's what I've been missing!" But what I've learned is that chasing squirrels keeps you moving but never arriving. It's exhausting.

I remember one morning vividly. I was at the gym, ready for another meticulously planned workout. My notebook was open—reps, sets, rest times, all laid out in a green hardcover notebook. (We didn't have apps to track those things yet.) My heart-rate monitor was strapped around my chest. My mini disc player was loaded with my "mixed tape." Everything was in its place, according to plan. Except this time it didn't feel right.

I felt totally disconnected from my body, unable to focus because of an article I read about "metabolic confusion" (hello, squirrel #87), knowing I should tweak my macros, or revise my workout split. I wasn't in my body—I was in my head, chasing squirrels. That's when I realized I wasn't doing any of this because I wanted to. I was doing it out of fear. Fear of falling behind. Fear of not doing enough. Fear of getting it wrong.

So, I did something radical.
I closed the notebook.
I unstrapped my heart rate monitor.
And I just moved.
No rep counting.
No comparing.
Just me–and Cher singing 'Believe" on my mini disk player.

For the first time in a long time, I felt my body again. And that's when the language in my head began to change. As I left the gym, "Did I do enough?" became "How did that feel?"

These days, as I prepare to work out, I'll ask myself, "What do I need today?" Not what do I need to do or what should I do, just what do I need? I also ask "what sounds good?" "What sounds fun?"

Some days, it's a heavy lifting session. Some days, it's a walk with my chihuahua, Percy, and Stephen King. And some days, it's rest. My goal has shifted from perfection to connection to myself. If you feel caught up in The Squirrel Effect—the endless scrolling, comparing, tweaking, overthinking—I want you to know you can step away. When you stop chasing squirrels, they'll stop chasing you—with their bitty little attention spans, they won't even notice you're gone!

Now, when I catch sight of a squirrel out of the corner of my eye, I can smile and say, "cut, but no thanks." I've got better things to do. Feel the sun on my face. Breathe. Move because I get to, not because I have to.

That's what I hope this book got you closer to, and you're well on your way. You've got this!

References

Chapter 2: Menopause

Ajdžanovic, V. Z., Trifunovic, S., Miljic, D., Šošic-Jurjevic, B., Filipovic, B., Miler, M., Ristic, N., Manojlovic-Stojanoski, M., & Miloševic, V. (2018). Somatopause, weaknesses of the therapeutic approaches and the cautious optimism based on experimental ageing studies with soy isoflavones. *EXCLI journal, 17*, 279–301. https://doi.org/10.17179/excli2017-956

Avis NE, Crawford SL, Greendale G, Bromberger JT, Everson-Rose SA, Gold EB, Hess R, Joffe H, Kravitz HM, Tepper PG, Thurston RC; Study of Women's Health Across the Nation. Duration of menopausal vasomotor symptoms over the menopause transition. JAMA Intern Med. 2015 Apr;175(4):531-9. doi: 10.1001/jamainternmed.2014.8063. PMID: 25686030; PMCID: PMC4433164.

El Khoudary SR, Aggarwal B, Beckie TM, Hodis HN, Johnson AE, Langer RD, Limacher MC, Manson JE, Stefanick ML, Allison MA; American Heart Association Prevention Science Committee of the Council on Epidemiology and Prevention; and Council on Cardiovascular and Stroke Nursing. Menopause Transition and Cardiovascular Disease Risk: Implications for Timing of Early Prevention: A Scientific Statement From the American Heart Association. Circulation. 2020 Dec 22;142(25):e506-e532. doi: 10.1161/CIR.0000000000000912. Epub 2020 Nov 30. PMID: 33251828.

Faubion, Stephanie S. MD, MBA, FACP, NCMP; Crandall, Carolyn J. MD, MS, MACP, NCMP, FASBMR; Davis, Lori DNP, FNP-C, NCMP; El Khoudary, Samar R. PhD, MPH, FAHA; Hodis, Howard N. MD; Lobo, Roger A. MD; Maki, Pauline M. PhD; Manson, JoAnn E. MD, DrPH, MACP, NCMP; Pinkerton, JoAnn V. MD, FACOG, NCMP; Santoro, Nanette F. MD; Shifren, Jan L. MD, NCMP; Shufelt, Chrisandra L. MD, MS, FACP, NCMP; Thurston,

Rebecca C. PhD, FABMR, FAPS; Wolfman, Wendy MD, FRCSC, FACOG. The 2022 hormone therapy position statement of The North American Menopause Society. Menopause 29(7):p 767-794, July 2022. | DOI: 10.1097/GME.0000000000002028

Freeman, E. W., Sammel, M. D., & Sanders, R. J. (2014). Risk of long-term hot flashes after natural menopause: evidence from the Penn Ovarian Aging Study cohort. *Menopause (New York, N.Y.), 21*(9), 924–932. https://doi.org/10.1097/GME.0000000000000196

Hall J. E. (2015). Endocrinology of the Menopause. *Endocrinology and metabolism clinics of North America, 44*(3), 485–496. https://doi.org/10.1016/j.ecl.2015.05.010

Herrera, A. Y., Hodis, H. N., Mack, W. J., & Mather, M. (2017). Estradiol Therapy After Menopause Mitigates Effects of Stress on Cortisol and Working Memory. *The Journal of clinical endocrinology and metabolism, 102*(12), 4457–4466. https://doi.org/10.1210/jc.2017-00825

Hershner, S., & O'Brien, L. M. (2018). The Impact of a Randomized Sleep Education Intervention for College Students. *Journal of clinical sleep medicine : JCSM : official publication of the American Academy of Sleep Medicine, 14*(3), 337–347. https://doi.org/10.5664/jcsm.6974

Motlani, V., Motlani, G., Pamnani, S., Sahu, A., & Acharya, N. (2023). Endocrine Changes in Postmenopausal Women: A Comprehensive View. *Cureus, 15*(12), e51287. https://doi.org/10.7759/cureus.51287

Raloff, J. (November, 2017). Explainer: What is a hormone? https://www.snexplores.org/article/explainer-what-hormone

Rossman J. (2019). Cognitive-Behavioral Therapy for Insomnia: An Effective and Underutilized Treatment for Insomnia. *American journal of lifestyle medicine, 13*(6), 544–547. https://doi.org/10.1177/1559827619867677

Rossouw JE, Anderson GL, Prentice RL, et al. *Risks and benefits of estrogen plus progestin in healthy postmenopausal women: principal results from the Women's Health Initiative randomized controlled trial.* JAMA. 2002;288(3):321-33. doi:10.1001/jama.288.3.321

Soares, Claudio N. MD, PhD, FRCPC, MBA(c). Mood disorders in midlife women: understanding the critical window and its clinical implications. Menopause 21(2):p 198-206, February 2014. | DOI: 10.1097/GME.0000000000000193

Sutton-Tyrrell, Kim, Selzer, Faith, Sowers, MaryFran R. (Mary Francis Roy), Finkelstein, Joel S., Powell, Lynda H., Gold, Ellen B., . . . Matthews, Karen A. Study of Women's Health Across the Nation (SWAN), 2002-2004: Visit 06 Dataset. Inter-university Consortium for Political and Social Research [distributor], 2025-06-30. https://doi.org/10.3886/ICPSR31181.v3

Walker, J., Muench, A., Perlis, M. L., & Vargas, I. (2022). Cognitive Behavioral Therapy for Insomnia (CBT-I): A Primer. *Klinicheskaia i spetsial'naia psikhologiia = Clinical psychology and special education*, *11*(2), 123–137. https://doi.org/10.17759/cpse.2022110208

Wright VJ, Schwartzman JD, Itinoche R, Wittstein J. The musculoskeletal syndrome of menopause. Climacteric. 2024 Oct;27(5):466-472. doi: 10.1080/13697137.2024.2380363. Epub 2024 Jul 30. PMID: 39077777.

Chapter 3: Who The Hell Am I Now?

Break Binge Eating (2024) Body Image Statistics 2024 57+ Shocking Facts & Stats https://breakbingeeating.com/body-image-statistics/

Medeiros de Morais, M. S., Macêdo, S. G. G. F., do Nascimento, R. A., Vieira, M. C. A., Moreira, M. A., da Câmara, S. M. A., Almeida, M. D. G., & Maciel, Á. C. C. (2024). Dissatisfaction with body image and weight gain in middle-aged women:

A cross sectional study. *PloS one, 19*(1), e0290380. https://doi.org/10.1371/journal.pone.0290380

NOW Foundation (2025) Get The Facts. https://now.org/now-foundation/love-your-body/love-your-body-whats-it-all-about/get-the-facts/

Vendemia, Megan; Goodboy, A Alan K; Chiasson, Rebekah M ; Dillow, Megan R. Person-specific effects of women's social media use on body image concerns: an intensive longitudinal study of daily life, *Human Communication Research*, Volume 51, Issue 3, June 2025, Pages 164–178, https://doi.org/10.1093/hcr/hqaf001

Vincent C, Bodnaruc AM, Prud'homme D, Olson V, Giroux I. Associations between menopause and body image: A systematic review. *Women's Health*. 2023;19. doi:10.1177/17455057231209536

Williams L, Gurung J, Persons P, Kilpela L. Body image and eating issues in midlife: A narrative review with clinical question recommendations. Maturitas. 2024 Oct;188:108068. doi: 10.1016/j.maturitas.2024.108068. Epub 2024 Jul 20. PMID: 39084135; PMCID: PMC12186726.

Chapter 4: Body Image

Baceviciene, M., Jankauskiene, R., & Swami, V. (2021). Nature Exposure and Positive Body Image: A Cross-Sectional Study Examining the Mediating Roles of Physical Activity, Autonomous Motivation, Connectedness to Nature, and Perceived Restorativeness. *International journal of environmental research and public health*, *18*(22), 12246. https://doi.org/10.3390/ijerph182212246

Teas J, Hurley T, Msph SG, Mph KO. Walking outside Improves Mood for Healthy Postmenopausal Women. *Clinical medicine Oncology*. 2007;1. doi:10.4137/CMO.S343

Chapter 5 & 6: Move Through Menopause and Designing Your Movement Map

Abiç A, Yilmaz Vefikuluçay D. The Effect of Yoga on Menopause Symptoms: A Randomized Controlled Trial. Holist Nurs Pract. 2024 May-Jun 01;38(3):138-147. doi: 10.1097/HNP.0000000000000646. Epub 2024 May 6. PMID: 38709129.

Atakan, M. M., Li, Y., Koşar, Ş. N., Turnagöl, H. H., & Yan, X. (2021). Evidence-Based Effects of High-Intensity Interval Training on Exercise Capacity and Health: A Review with Historical Perspective. *International journal of environmental research and public health, 18*(13), 7201. https://doi.org/10.3390/ijerph18137201

Basat H, Esmaeilzadeh S, Eskiyurt N. The effects of strengthening and high-impact exercises on bone metabolism and quality of life in postmenopausal women: a randomized controlled trial. J Back Musculoskelet Rehabil. 2013;26(4):427-35. doi: 10.3233/BMR-130402. PMID: 23948830.

Berin E, Hammar M, Lindblom H, Lindh-Åstrand L, Rubér M, Spetz Holm AC. Resistance training for hot flushes in postmenopausal women: A randomised controlled trial. Maturitas. 2019 Aug;126:55-60. doi: 10.1016/j.maturitas.2019.05.005. Epub 2019 May 14. PMID: 31239119.

Boutcher, Yati N.; Boutcher, Stephen H.; Yoo, Hye; Meerkin, Jarrod D.. The Effect of Sprint Interval Training on Body Composition of Postmenopausal Women. Medicine & Science in Sports & Exercise 51(7):p 1413-1419, July 2019. | DOI: 10.1249/MSS.0000000000001919

Chang, X., Xu, S., & Zhang, H. (2022). Regulation of bone health through physical exercise: Mechanisms and types. *Frontiers in endocrinology, 13*, 1029475. https://doi.org/10.3389/fendo.2022.1029475

Cramer, H., Lauche, R., Langhorst, J., & Dobos, G. (2012). Effectiveness of yoga for menopausal symptoms: a systematic review and meta-analysis of randomized controlled trials. *Evidence-based complementary and alternative medicine : eCAM*, *2012*, 863905. https://doi.org/10.1155/2012/863905

Dias, R.K.N., Penna, E.M., Noronha, Á.S.N. et al. Minimal dose resistance training enhances strength without affecting cardiac autonomic modulation in menopausal women: a randomized clinical trial. Sci Rep 14, 19355 (2024). https://doi.org/10.1038/s41598-024-69073-4

Dupuit M, Maillard F, Pereira B, Marquezi ML, Lancha AH Jr, Boisseau N. Effect of high intensity interval training on body composition in women before and after menopause: a meta-analysis. Exp Physiol. 2020 Sep;105(9):1470-1490. doi: 10.1113/EP088654. Epub 2020 Jul 21. PMID: 32613697.

Elavsky S. (2009). Physical activity, menopause, and quality of life: the role of affect and self-worth across time. *Menopause (New York, N.Y.)*, *16*(2), 265–271. https://doi.org/10.1097/gme.0b013e31818c0284

Guadalupe-Grau A, Fuentes T, Guerra B, Calbet JA. Exercise and bone mass in adults. Sports Med. 2009;39(6):439-68. doi: 10.2165/00007256-200939060-00002. PMID: 19453205.

Iwata, M., Yamamoto, A., Matsuo, S., Hatano, G., Miyazaki, M., Fukaya, T., Fujiwara, M., Asai, Y., & Suzuki, S. (2019). Dynamic Stretching Has Sustained Effects on Range of Motion and Passive Stiffness of the Hamstring Muscles. *Journal of sports science & medicine*, *18*(1), 13–20.

Jorge MP, Santaella DF, Pontes IM, Shiramizu VK, Nascimento EB, Cabral A, Lemos TM, Silva RH, Ribeiro AM. Hatha Yoga practice decreases menopause symptoms and improves quality of life: A randomized controlled trial. Complement Ther Med. 2016 Jun;26:128-35. doi: 10.1016/j.ctim.2016.03.014. Epub 2016 Mar 22. PMID: 27261993.

Konrad A, Tilp M and Nakamura M (2021) A Comparison of the Effects of Foam Rolling and Stretching on Physical Performance. A Systematic Review and Meta-Analysis. *Front. Physiol.* 12:720531. doi: 10.3389/fphys.2021.720531

Kurt, C., Gürol, B., & Nebioğlu, İ. Ö. (2023). Effects of traditional stretching versus self-myofascial release warm-up on physical performance in well-trained female athletes. *Journal of musculoskeletal & neuronal interactions*, *23*(1), 61–71.

Lv, Y., & Yin, Y. (2024). A Review of the Application of Myofascial Release Therapy in the Treatment of Diseases. *Journal of multidisciplinary healthcare*, *17*, 4507–4517. https://doi.org/10.2147/JMDH.S481706

Maddalozzo GF, Widrick JJ, Cardinal BJ, Winters-Stone KM, Hoffman MA, Snow CM. The effects of hormone replacement therapy and resistance training on spine bone mineral density in early postmenopausal women. Bone. 2007 May;40(5):1244-51. doi: 10.1016/j.bone.2006.12.059. Epub 2006 Dec 29. PMID: 17291843.

Manaye, S., Cheran, K., Murthy, C., Bornemann, E. A., Kamma, H. K., Alabbas, M., Elashahab, M., Abid, N., & Arcia Franchini, A. P. (2023). The Role of High-intensity and High-impact Exercises in Improving Bone Health in Postmenopausal Women: A Systematic Review. *Cureus*, *15*(2), e34644. https://doi.org/10.7759/cureus.34644

Ng CA, Gandham A, Mesinovic J, Owen PJ, Ebeling PR, Scott D. Effects of Moderate-to High-Impact Exercise Training on Bone Structure Across the Lifespan: A Systematic Review and Meta-Analysis of Randomized Controlled Trials. J Bone Miner Res. 2023 Nov;38(11):1612-1634. doi: 10.1002/jbmr.4899. Epub 2023 Sep 4. PMID: 37555459.

Nichol, L.; Battey, G.; Mitchell, S.; Shibata, T.; and Witzke, FACSM, K. (2017) "Effects on Dynamic and Static Stretching and Self-Myofascial Release on Muscle Power and Flexibility." *International Journal of Exercise Science: Conference Proceedings*:

Vol. 8: Iss. 5, Article 51.https://digitalcommons.wku.edu/ijesab/vol8/iss5/51

Papadakis G, Hans D, Gonzalez-Rodriguez E, Vollenweider P, Waeber G, Marques-Vidal PM, Lamy O. The Benefit of Menopausal Hormone Therapy on Bone Density and Microarchitecture Persists After its Withdrawal. J Clin Endocrinol Metab. 2016 Dec;101(12):5004-5011. doi: 10.1210/jc.2016-2695. Epub 2016 Nov 17. PMID: 27854548.

Platt O, Bateman J, Bakour S. Impact of menopause hormone therapy, exercise, and their combination on bone mineral density and mental wellbeing in menopausal women: a scoping review. Front Reprod Health. 2025 May 12;7:1542746. doi: 10.3389/frph.2025.1542746. PMID: 40421002; PMCID: PMC12104296.

SEER Training Modules, *Module Name*. U. S. National Institutes of Health, National Cancer Institute. (November, 2025) https://training.seer.cancer.gov/anatomy/skeletal/growth.html

Silva, B. C., & Hipólito Rodrigues, M. A. (2023). Estrogen hormone therapy and postmenopausal osteoporosis: does it really take two to tango? *Women & Health, 63*(10), 770–773. https://doi.org/10.1080/03630242.2023.2278211

Wang Y, Shan W, Li Q, Yang N, Shan W. Tai Chi Exercise for the Quality of Life in a Perimenopausal Women Organization: A Systematic Review. Worldviews Evid Based Nurs. 2017 Aug;14(4):294-305. doi: 10.1111/wvn.12234. Erratum in: Worldviews Evid Based Nurs. 2017 Oct;14(5):424. doi: 10.1111/wvn.12256. PMID: 28742289.

Watson SL, Weeks BK, Weis LJ, Harding AT, Horan SA, Beck BR. High-Intensity Resistance and Impact Training Improves Bone Mineral Density and Physical Function in Postmenopausal Women With Osteopenia and Osteoporosis: The LIFTMOR Randomized Controlled Trial. J Bone Miner Res. 2018 Feb;33(2):211-220. doi: 10.1002/jbmr.3284. Epub 2017 Oct 4. Erratum in: J Bone Miner Res. 2019 Mar;34(3):572. doi: 10.1002/jbmr.3659. PMID: 28975661.

Warneke, Konstantin; Wirth, Klaus; Keiner, Michael; and Schiemann, Stephan (2023) "Improvements in flexibility depending on stretching duration," *International Journal of Exercise Science*: Vol. 16 : Iss. 4, Pages 83 - 94. DOI: https://doi.org/10.70252/LBOU2008

Chapter 7: Motivation

Milkman, Katherine (2017). Why we fail and how we stand up afterwards. TEDxPenn. https://www.youtube.com/watch?v=zaf3yQ4OLdw

Chapter 8: Nourishment

Hall, K. D., & Kahan, S. (2018). Maintenance of Lost Weight and Long-Term Management of Obesity. *The Medical clinics of North America, 102*(1), 183–197. https://doi.org/10.1016/j.mcna.2017.08.012

Ismaiel, A., Scarlata, G.G.M., Boitos, I. *et al.* Gastrointestinal adverse events associated with GLP-1 RA in non-diabetic patients with overweight or obesity: a systematic review and network meta-analysis. *Int J Obes* 49, 1946–1957 (2025). https://doi.org/10.1038/s41366-025-01859-6

Moll H, Frey E, Gerber P, Geidl B, Kaufmann M, Braun J, Beuschlein F, Puhan MA, Yebyo HG. GLP-1 receptor agonists for weight reduction in people living with obesity but without diabetes: a living benefit-harm modelling study. EClinicalMedicine. 2024 May 27;73:102661. doi: 10.1016/j.eclinm.2024.102661. PMID: 38846069; PMCID: PMC11154119.

Pélissier L, Bagot S, Miles-Chan JL, Pereira B, Boirie Y, Duclos M, Dulloo A, Isacco L, Thivel D. Is dieting a risk for higher weight gain in normal-weight individual? A systematic review and meta-analysis. Br J Nutr. 2023 Oct 14;130(7):1190-1212. doi: 10.1017/S0007114523000132. Epub 2023 Jan 16. PMID: 36645258.

Sweatt, K., Garvey, W. T., & Martins, C. (2024). Strengths and Limitations of BMI in the Diagnosis of Obesity: What is the Path Forward?. *Current obesity reports, 13*(3), 584–595. https://doi.org/10.1007/s13679-024-00580-1

Tylka, T. L., Annunziato, R. A., Burgard, D., Daníelsdóttir, S., Shuman, E., Davis, C., & Calogero, R. M. (2014). The weight-inclusive versus weight-normative approach to health: evaluating the evidence for prioritizing well-being over weight loss. *Journal of obesity, 2014*, 983495. https://doi.org/10.1155/2014/983495

www.ingramcontent.com/pod-product-compliance
Lightning Source LLC
Chambersburg PA
CBHW041831110726
48006CB00020B/2585